Meaningful Motion:
Biomechanics for Occupational Therapists

For Churchill Livingstone:

Commissioning editor: Susan Young
Development editor: Catherine Jackson
Production manager: Andrew Palfreyman
Designer: Keith Kail.

Meaningful Motion: Biomechanics for Occupational Therapists

Sandi J. Spaulding Ph.D, M.Sc., B.Sc. (OT), OT(C)

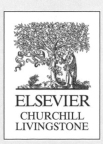

ELSEVIER
CHURCHILL
LIVINGSTONE

EDINBURGH LONDON NEW YORK OXFORD PHILADELPHIA ST LOUIS SYDNEY TORONTO 2005

ELSEVIER
CHURCHILL
LIVINGSTONE

An imprint of Elsevier Limited

© 2005, Elsevier Ltd
First published 2005

ISBN 0 443 07439 9

British Library Cataloguing in Publication Data
A catalogue record for this book is available from the British Library.

Library of Congress Cataloging in Publication Data
A catalog record for this book is available from the Library of Congress.

Note

Knowledge and best practice in this field are constantly changing. As new research and experience broaden our knowledge, changes in practice, treatment and drug therapy may become necessary or appropriate. Readers are advised to check the most current information provided (i) on procedures featured or (ii) by the manufacturer of each product to be administered, to verify the recommended dose or formula, the method and duration of administration, and contraindications. It is the responsibility of the practitioner, relying on their own experience and knowledge of the patient, to make diagnoses, to determine dosages and the best treatment for each individual patient, and to take all appropriate safety precautions.
To the fullest extent of the law, neither the publisher nor the authors assumes any liability for any injury and/or damage.

Printed in China

The Publisher's Policy is to use Paper manufactured from sustainable forests.

Contents

FOREWORD

Universities are changing in the way students are prepared. Greater emphasis is being place on interdisciplinary programs of study where students glean and extend the knowledge from a variety of different academic disciplines. Interdisciplinary research programs are being conducted by our professors, often in response to the funding criteria that agencies have established in recognition of the value of interdisciplinary research.

Professional practice in the health case sector is also travelling done a similar path. Interprofessional education programs are gaining momentum in our educational institutions and in the fields of practice. Health care administrators and professionals are seeing the value of addressing heath care issues from a number of professional perspectives like medicine, nursing, occupational therapy, physical therapy and social work to name but a few. We are witnessing the synergy that can transpire when traditional approaches to health care are augmented by the interventions from other professions. It is predicted that interprofessional education programs will a more regularized approach to effectively preparing health care professionals and delivering health care program.

Sandi Spaulding has extended this trend in the pages of her new book entitled *Meaningful Motion: Biomechanics for Occupational Therapists*. Spaulding summarizes the most recent and seminal research findings in the areas of biomechanics, motor control and behaviour and human movement science and she has effectively applied these concepts to the field of Occupational Therapy. Students, professors and clinicians will find the contents of this book invaluable to broadening their understandings, enriching their preparation, and advancing their practice. It aligns perfectly with the direction taken by both universities and professional practice.

Authors who write for multiple audiences run the risk of not reaching or losing some or all of the targeted groups. Furthermore, academics are frequently and many times, justifiably, criticized for writing books that do not reach the practitioner, and therefore do not inform or impact practice. Critics state, usually with compelling evidence, that academics speak in esoteric terms, and often speak exclusively and extensively to one another. Some of my professional friends accuse me and my academic colleagues of going to extreme and convoluted ends to explain the obvious. I believe that this is a fair, but unfortunate criticism.

Prolific academics like Henry Mintzberg from McGill University have entered the discussion by stating that academics often fail their fields of study and professions by not ensuring that their work is transferred to the front lines of practice. He claims that if academics are not effectively serving practitioners, then they are not effectively serving their disciplines/professions. While this is a strong statement, it is one with which I often agree. I have also been critical of myself and my colleagues for not ensuring that the implications of our work are clearly outlined and effectively shared with end users with a goal to more effectively inform practice. We often say that we will do something about this, but when it is all said and done, more is said than done.

Critics will have a hard time finding fault in Sandi Spaulding's new book - *Meaningful Motion:*

Biomechanics for Occupational Therapists. Spaulding effectively communicates to students, professors and practitioners alike, and members of all groups can gain valuable insights from digesting this book. Spaulding effectively blends theory and practice in the text by beginning each chapter with a case study to provide context to the theoretical material presented for the reader. After a through theoretical grounding in each of the key concepts, readers are presented with a series of questions related to the case study, and a concluding laboratory exercise to help encourage "praxis", or learning by doing.

I won't attempt to summarize what is in the book as this is not the purpose of a foreword. I can say as a kinesiology professor and university administrator for nearly 20 years, I have gained an appreciation for, and understanding of, the key contributors to the fields of biomechanics, motor control ergonomics and human movement science. The seminal works in these fields are cited in this text. Students from both kinesiology and occupational therapy will be well served by reading these chapters. As an educator I can also identify work that students will understand and apply. Spaulding has made this difficult and critical task an easy one for readers through her fluid writing style and the inclusion of valuable applied learning activities.

Finally, as a Dean of Health Sciences, I'm amazed by the overlap and synergy that can take place when students, academics and professionals engage in interdisciplinary and interprofessional research, study and practice. Sandi Spaulding has done a remarkable job of integrating the work from a number of fields and drawn significant application to the study and practice of occupational therapy.

Meaningful Motion will be a **meaningful** contribution to the academy and profession of occupational therapy. I'm pleased and honoured to be associated with this fine contribution to the literature.

W. James Weese, Ph.D
Professor and Dean
Faculty of Health Sciences
The University of Western Ontario

April, 2005

PREFACE

This textbook is about kinesiology principles for occupational therapy students and practising therapists. The book evolved through a need expressed by members of the occupational therapy community for a book they could use which incorporated both fields. There has been a concern by some occupational therapists and students that there is a great deal known about human movement but the knowledge has not always reached therapists in a way they can use it. Therapists are also finding that their co-workers, the individuals with whom they work, and their families want to know the basis for treatment techniques. This text is written to address those needs. It has been written specifically for members of the occupational therapy community. It is primarily for use by occupational therapy students, but it can also give experienced therapists new ways to help people who have movement difficulties.

The book is divided into nine chapters and separated into two sections. After the introduction, the first section explains some of the biomechanical and motor control principles which the reader will find useful in occupational therapy work. The second section discusses specific areas in which therapists work: balance training, the environment, ergonomics and leisure. The information from the first five chapters is integrated into these areas. The list of areas is by no means exhaustive, but will provide the reader with thorough examples of movement science applied to occupational therapy.

Each chapter begins with a comprehensive fictional case study. The case study is followed by specific principles of human movement based on knowledge and research about human movement. Within this section of each chapter there are many occupational therapy examples of the principles. The end of each chapter includes questions about the case. The person reading the chapter should be able to answer the questions based on the material in the chapter. Following the questions, there is either a laboratory exercise or a list of questions related to the material in the chapter. These exercises are designed to give the reader an opportunity to think further about the material in the chapter.

The overriding goal of writing this book was to introduce biomechanical and motor control and learning. It is hoped that the reader, once finished the book, will be able to apply these principles to practice. It is also hoped that the individuals with whom the reader works will be helped to be engaged more meaningfully in the occupations they want to undertake.

ACKNOWLEDGEMENTS

Many people have supported me through the process of compiling information and writing this book. These people included Lynda Weston, Pamela Houghton, Janet Brown, Marilyn Kertoy, Joyce MacKinnon, Marion Barnes, John Simmons, Maggie Reynolds, Kris Kobler, Chris Morgan, Thelma Sumsion, Joanne Cook, Sandra Hobson, Rothea Olivier, Christine Young, Joey Farrell and Linda Roe. Thanks also go to my colleagues at the University of Western Ontario for their support.

Frank Stein and Jim McPherson encouraged me to start this project and had faith that I would complete it. Doris Miller provided valuable support, encouragement and professional insight into the biomechanical concepts, the teaching principles, and the writing process throughout the project. I could not have finished it without her. Barbara Sexton was instrumental in encouraging me to forge ahead with the project. Unfortunately, she passed away before I had the opportunity to thank her.

A special thanks to Thelma Sumsion who encouraged me to take the time to write.

I want to thank Lynn Shaw, Lisa Klinger, Flora Stephenson, Paula Gilmore and Beata Batorowicz for kindly and thoughtfully reviewing preliminary chapters of the book. Ann Zilberbrant and Leann Merla provided excellent preliminary artwork for the illustrations. Lynda Weston edited the text thoroughly and professionally.

Lynn Shaw co-authored the chapter on ergonomics with me. I am grateful for her excellent input and enthusiasm. She added important information to that chapter. Any omissions or errors in the chapter are my responsibility, not Lynn's.

Wonderful interactions with people from different places reminded me that an understanding of cultural diversity is important for occupational therapists. We need to remember the diversity of people, even when we are discussing a topic as minimally related to culture as human motion would seem to be. Thanks to Averil Stewart, Ruth Watson, Rothea Olivier, Chris Olivier, Colla Swart, Freeman Patterson, André Gallant, Jennifer Wright, Lisa Klinger, Beata Batorowicz and Flora Stephenson. All of these people, in their own ways, kept me cognisant of the need to think about cultural, community and individual values as I produced this text.

I am grateful to the students whom I have taught over the years at the University of Indianapolis, the University of Wisconsin-Milwaukee, and the University of Western Ontario. They showed enthusiasm, wanted to become better therapists, and asked me thoughtful and important questions. I want to thank these students because their desire for the information in this book is truly the reason it has been written.

I wish to acknowledge important financial support in the form of an author's grant I received from the Canadian Association of Occupational Therapists.

My family members, including Trish, Brenda and Neil Spaulding, Jessica and Miranda Burley, John and Helen Pinel, and my daughter, Carly, were all there for me. Thank you

DEDICATION

This book is dedicated in loving memory to my father, John Hanna Spaulding, BASc, PEng. He taught me physics and mechanics creatively. His teaching made me realise these were disciplines with applications to my interest in human motion. I would not have chosen this road without him.

Chapter 1

Introduction

Many occupational therapy students express frustration when they are learning about human motion. They say there is no reason for occupational therapists to learn about biomechanics. Sometimes they also express disappointment because there are no detailed biomechanics books designed specifically for them. They want a book that gives them examples of how they can use the science of motion. They do not want to guess about occupational therapy applications or extrapolate ideas from sports or physical therapy books. It is not surprising that without textbooks that directly address their issues, they do not think studying motion is important for them. This book will equip them with the ability to do therapy with their clients who have physical problems.

This book is designed for these occupational therapy students and occupational therapists. It is a book written specifically for occupational therapy practice. The fictional cases relate to individual-centred occupational issues. The examples are ones therapists can understand. The laboratory exercises are designed to provide insight into motion for occupational therapy students. Some of the exercises provide information about the difficulties the individuals they work with will face. Other exercises provide occupational therapy professionals with ideas to incorporate into their treatment plans.

So often when therapists describe to me how they have solved problems during therapeutic interventions, I am made acutely aware that they have intuitively used mechanical principles. This text will help them frame that intuition. They can move forward with renewed confidence in applying and expanding their use of principles of human motion.

CLINICAL BIOMECHANICS AND ITS RELATION TO OCCUPATIONS

The book is in two sections although there is some overlap. The first section addresses some of the principles of human motion science and the second part applies some of those concepts to areas of occupational therapy. The book begins with chapters addressing specific biomechanical principles including kinematics, kinetics and mechanical principles in the second, third and fourth chapters.

The fifth chapter is also one that addresses principles of human motion science, specifically motor control and motor learning principles. The concepts in this fifth chapter are based on the specialty of kinesiology that is often referred to as psychomotor control. This section is included because the area of study describes how people teach and learn human movement. Occupational therapists teach motion and the individuals they work with try to control and learn movements. This teaching and learning happens so frequently in our therapy. The application of psychomotor control principles will enhance many therapeutic interventions with people who have physical problems.

The last chapters address specific issues including balance, the environment, work and leisure. These chapters are designed to help the therapist see how principles of human movement are being researched and used. The chapters will help them apply the principles to their own practices.

Issues addressed through biomechanics research

Biomechanics researchers and kinesiology (the area of study of which biomechanics is one specialty) researchers have addressed many movement issues that arise for people with physical problems. There is a good history of research in many areas including balance, leisure and ergonomics. The results of this relevant research are addressed in this text. Readers are urged to do more reading in the research areas that apply to their areas of practice. It is exciting to see research that incorporates the principles of kinesiology with occupational therapy. I think our treatment can only improve as we learn more about how to frame some of it using the concepts and research of clinical kinesiology.

Quantitative and qualitative problems

Most occupational therapists do not have access to extensive biomechanics equipment. Even if therapists did have access to the equipment and techniques, biomechanical analyses would require more time than would be feasible for therapists to use. Therapists also work with people who have complex movement patterns and these movements are difficult to evaluate with biomechanical equipment. Most of the problems and exercises in the text are of a qualitative nature. This means the ideas can be used without relying on biomechanics equipment and complex mathematical calculations. The content of the chapters, however, does use some of the quantitative information that is available to biomechanists. The approach is qualitative only in the context of biomechanics.

Problem-solving approach

Each chapter in the text has a case associated with it. These cases are presented at the beginning of each chapter so that the reader will have an idea of an individual who may be helped through applying some of the concepts of the chapter. I recommend that the reader thoroughly understand the case at the beginning of the chapter. There are questions at the end of the chapter, related to the case. The reader can consider how the principles and research described in the chapter could be applied to the person in the case. The cases are fictional composites of individuals with physical problems, and therefore represent people similar to those with whom occupational therapists work.

The following case study can be reviewed as the reader works through the text. By the end of the book, the reader should have ideas to help Ms Andrews, based on the material in it.

CASE STUDY: MS MEREDITH ANDREWS

Ms Meredith Andrews is a 37-year-old woman who lives in a large urban area. She has a very full and active professional and personal life. She has managed this life while dealing with the effects of limb-girdle muscular dystrophy, with which she was diagnosed when she was 7 years old.

She is a computer hardware designer in a centre for children who need computer technology to communicate with others. She enjoys the work tremendously. She gets personal satisfaction from working with the children and therapists in the centre. She thrives on problem-solving and designing complex equipment that the children can then use in their everyday lives.

Ms Andrews has not been totally satisfied with her level of computer hardware knowledge and is intent on learning more about computer hardware design. To fulfil this need to study, she decided to work part-time on a doctorate degree in hardware technology at a large urban university setting. She has done this while cutting back on her work hours, so she is working about 15 hours a week.

She has finished her course work and comprehensive exams in her PhD programme. She is now conducting her doctoral research on the use of a new head movement operated switch mechanism she designed for children with cerebral palsy who have head control, but lack other voluntary movements. Her data collection is going well.

In her leisure time, she and her husband relish travelling. They have been to Hong Kong, New Zealand and Morocco in the last three years. She has been able to adapt whatever she needs, so that travel is not only possible, but very enjoyable.

She is finding that she is beginning to have physical difficulties that are impeding her ability to participate in her chosen lifestyle. She is starting to have difficulties conducting her work activities of constructing and installing the equipment. Her proximal musculature weakness seems to have increased in the last year to a point where she has difficulty accommodating to it, both in her work environments and in all other aspects of her life.

The setting

There are a number of settings which are starting to pose problems for Ms Andrews. One setting is her home. She is involved in maintaining her home and participating in family activities. She and her husband do not have children, but she has four siblings and her husband has five. They have many nieces and nephews whom they enjoy greatly. The families all live fairly close together, so it is a rare weekend that Ms Andrews and her husband do not have the opportunity of spending time with members of their extended family.

The second setting is her academic environment, which is a university setting where she is conducting her doctoral thesis. She is testing the head control system to see if it is effective for children in the treatment centre in which she works. The laboratory in which she works is at the back of a large building and even getting to the room is beginning to be tiring.

The third environment consists of transportation and travel. Her travelling is beginning to be difficult because of her lack of strength in both her shoulders and her hips.

The occupational therapist

Ms Margot McAllister has been involved with Ms Andrews and her family off and on as the disease has slowly progressed, when Ms Andrews has particular issues. At this point in time Ms McAllister has a number of years of experience working with adults in an outpatient setting that is designed to help people who have neuromuscular problems, such as those of Ms Andrews.

The individual

Ms Andrews is concerned about her physical limitations. These difficulties would be expected in someone who has limb-girdle muscular dystrophy. She has a very active lifestyle and this is overwhelming her at this time.

Physical abilities

Ms Andrews has decreased strength in both her shoulder girdle and hip musculature. She has enough strength to lift small objects with her arms. She cannot lift anything over 5 kg. She can walk, but finds that it is becoming tiring to go any distance over about 100 m. Her hip musculature is not strong enough for her to go any further, particularly if the ground surfaces are rough or she needs to walk on hills, steps or ramps.

Emotional status

Ms Andrews has lived most of her life with this disability of limb-girdle muscular dystrophy. She understands that it is slowly progressive and has been able to accommodate her activities as her physical abilities change. She has come to terms with the disability, because it has not stopped her from pursuing activities.

She is, however, more frustrated and upset at this time than she has ever been in the past. Her feelings of dissatisfaction are not so much because of experiencing declining strength, but because this strength reduction is causing limitations in her life. She is doing so many things professionally that are important and satisfying to her, but she is very afraid that she may not be able to continue to do some of them. She is afraid that she may not be able to finish her degree and is frightened by the thought that she and her husband may have to stop travelling.

She really would like to continue her chosen occupations. She does not want even to think of giving up these occupations. She does not want to compromise her goals because of her disability.

Her husband has always been and continues to be very supportive. He knew that she had muscular dystrophy at the time of their marriage and he thought it was an issue with which they could cope. He is concerned now because his wife is stressed and seems to see the future as bleak.

Ms Andrews is further stressed because her time with her husband and family has decreased because of the demands of her doctoral work and her employment. She is not quite sure how to reconcile her work and her family life at this time, especially with the added burden of her ever-decreasing physical strength.

Exploring issues with Ms Andrews

The issues for Ms Andrews are extensive. She wants to complete her doctorate. She does not want to stop working. She also wants to continue to travel. She and her husband were hoping to tour the east coast of North America, including the eastern provinces of Canada and the eastern seaboard of the United States. She really thinks, though, that her life occupations, including travelling, seem to be falling outside her reach.

Her hope now rests with the occupational therapist who has helped her in the past. She has spoken with Ms McAllister over the phone and described some of her concerns and misgivings. Ms McAllister has set up a time to see her soon, so they can discuss the details of her concerns and address them.

Ms McAllister has her own concerns about the number of occupations in which Ms Andrews is engaged. She thinks that she and Ms Andrews will have to consider some major accommodations and adaptations of her occupations. She is not sure how well Ms Andrews will accept changes or contemplate reducing her expectations of herself. She will work with her client, though, to determine with her what can be done to help her.

QUESTIONS BASED ON THE CASE

Throughout this book, you will be provided with information about occupational therapy and biomechanics. Keep this person, Ms Andrews, in mind during your reading. You will be able to return to this case when you are finished the book and you will have specific recommendations for Ms Andrews.

While you are reading and studying the concepts in the book you might want to come back and consider her situation. Think about what some of the specific problems are for her. Are there changes you can recommend for her, based on biomechanics? What are the enablers of her occupations? What are the environmental demands? Would you recommend particular equipment or occupational changes? You can make assumptions about Ms Andrews's environments and lifestyles. Work towards solving some of her issues using your assumptions, the information provided in the case and the knowledge that you gain as you read.

SECTION 1

Principles of movement

Chapter 2

Occupational therapy and kinematics: how to describe occupations through movement

CHAPTER CONTENTS

Occupational therapists watch and try to change movement patterns every time they work with someone who has difficulty moving. The goals of treatment can range from trying to reduce the tremor of someone who has Parkinson's disease to strengthening someone's muscles who has sustained a spinal cord injury. These movements are done in the context of occupation, because the ultimate goal of being able to move is to do something with the movements. Movement is the basis of all physical occupations. The purpose of this chapter is to provide the occupational therapy student or practising therapist with definitions, concepts and tools to comprehend movement.

Understanding movement is crucial to effectively helping individuals with movement difficulties. If we do not understand some of the characteristics of movement, it is hard to explore the problems that movement difficulties create. When an occupational therapist works with an individual who has difficulty with movements, the therapist needs to understand the characteristics of the movements and how these actions impact occupations. The scientific literature that has been published about movements involved in occupations is becoming sophisticated and relevant. This research is exciting, because it is giving us new ways to approach our therapy and help our clients achieve their goals. We are only beginning to benefit from clinical biomechanics research. The knowledge provided to us by this research should continue and our ability to make use of it will also grow.

The students and therapists who understand the concepts of kinematics and movement will be able to improve their practice techniques when working with individuals. They will be able to do so because they will more readily see movement substitution (an awkward movement that occurs sometimes because the needed muscle force is absent). They will be able to document movement speed changes and other aspects of movement so they can better observe and document changes as treatment progresses. They can also understand the implications of adapting and accommodating movements more easily.

The description of the person in the following case is designed to address the issues of kinematics or the study of movements without having to consider the forces, such as muscle strength, producing those movements. Read the following case carefully and refer back to it as you go through the information in the chapter. There will be questions on the case at the end of the chapter, to help you understand and integrate concepts into your practice.

CASE STUDY: MR MARK DEGURSE

Mr Mark DeGurse is a 52-year-old married farmer. He and his wife have 5 children. Three of them, two boys and a girl, still live at home and contribute substantially to the work of the farm both after school in the winter and during the summer.

Mr DeGurse was injured in a farming accident, when he was trying to fix a piece of farm machinery in his cornfield while he was harvesting his corn in the autumn. He was by himself and decided to fix the equipment anyway, without waiting for help. It was an unfortunate decision, because he did not see a very heavy piece of the harvester above him loosen. This part of the harvester gave way and fell on his back. He was found by his teenage son about 2 hours later.

He was rushed to the closest community hospital, then because of the suspected severity of his injuries, he was airlifted to a large regional hospital. There it was determined that he had sustained internal injuries and a fracture of the third lumbar vertebra. He had surgery that successfully repaired the internal injuries. He was not as lucky with the fracture of his spine. His spinal cord was completely severed below the level of L_3, resulting in paraplegia.

Mr DeGurse spent 4 weeks in intensive care, then after 3 weeks in an acute medical care unit, he was transferred to the rehabilitation unit.

The setting

Mr DeGurse was airlifted to a large teaching hospital in a city approximately 200 km from his small farming community. The hospital specialised in emergency medicine and the acute care of individuals with internal, neurological and orthopaedic problems. The hospital had a large rehabilitation unit with therapists who worked with people who had been medically stabilized but needed extensive therapy before they either returned home or were found appropriate living accommodation. The rehabilitation department to which Mr DeGurse was transferred consisted of experienced occupational and physical therapists as well as other healthcare professionals, such as speech and language therapists, who were also necessary members of a full rehabilitation team.

The occupational therapist

Mr Matthew Parker was the occupational therapist who was going to work with Mr DeGurse while he was on the rehabilitation unit. Mr Parker had worked for 10 years in this rehabilitation unit with individuals who had sustained spinal cord injuries. He was considered to be an expert clinician by his colleagues in the city and had a senior therapist position as well as being a team leader for the rehabilitation unit. He was frequently asked to help other therapists and individuals who may have been having difficulty solving problems related to their rehabilitation. He was most experienced working with individuals who lived and worked in the large city and who had been injured in motor vehicle or industrial accidents.

He was comfortable working with Mr DeGurse and his injury, but was concerned at his own lack of understanding of the type of large family farm that Mr DeGurse and his wife owned and operated. This lack of knowledge was a problem, because he did not know how he was going to help Mr DeGurse make adaptations to his farm, so he could continue his work there. He was not even sure if it was possible to make enough accommodations and adaptations for Mr DeGurse to return to his work life.

The individual

Mr DeGurse, a man who knows about hard work, has spent his entire life farming in the Midwest of the United States. His parents immigrated there and started farming the land he now works, before he was born. He has a strong character and knows how to handle adversity but he has found the physical injury he has sustained much more difficult to deal with than anything he has experienced before in his life.

He knows that he will not be able to walk again. He has been in rehabilitation long enough with other people who also have spinal cord injuries to know he will also have other problems that seem insurmountable to him right now. He realises that he has a lot of work to do in rehabilitation before he can even consider whether he and his wife will be able to continue farming and carrying on their normal family life. He is not used to being in a hospital or being unable to take care of himself. He misses being with his wife and family on the farm that has always been part of his life.

Physical abilities

Mr DeGurse is severely limited right now due to the devastating effects of his spinal cord injury. He cannot take care of his own personal hygiene or do even simple activities such as dressing himself. He finds these limitations extraordinarily frustrating and expressed this when he first met with Mr. Parker.

He is also extremely upset because he really does not know if he will be able to continue on his farm and support his family financially. His family and farm mean everything to him and it is hard for him even to envision what the future might bring. He is not sure if his farm insurance will help with any of his costs.

The vertebral fracture that Mr DeGurse had has healed sufficiently for him to start into the rehabilitation process, but he is still very weak and fatigues easily. Even though the lesion did not interrupt nerve supply to his arms, he lacks his normal strength in his upper extremities.

He has been working on sitting balance during the acute phase of his rehabilitation. He can sit with back support for about 20 minutes before he fatigues completely and must return to sitting in a wheelchair or lie down in bed. He can feed himself, but even that seems an effort still. Other activities, let alone his former occupations, are beyond his abilities.

Emotional status

Mr DeGurse is very upset and depressed about his situation. He has very little idea of what the future holds for him. He has started working with the social worker and with Mr Parker to think about his future. They are trying to assure him that he will be able to return home and participate in many of his occupations. The therapists are trying to make contacts in the farming communities around the city and with other therapists to find another farmer who has sustained an injury who could talk with Mr DeGurse. They think meeting someone who has had a similar experience and has been able to return home with accommodations for the injury will make a big difference for Mr DeGurse's view of the future. They also hope that someone who is a farmer and does his work using a wheelchair will give them some ideas about what can be accomplished and what sort of adaptations they should be exploring with Mr DeGurse.

Mr DeGurse has many factors that are in his favour and will help him through the changes in his life his injury will make. He has a strong will. His wife is a good support and they have a stable relationship. His children have always been responsible on the farm, but they have never had to be a support to their father, so this injury has been very difficult for them to deal with and accept.

Mr DeGurse is devoted to his family. He is also an active leader in the community, particularly when it comes to helping his neighbours and planning recreational activities, such as children's baseball teams and other community events. He has good friends in the community. Many of his friends have taken the time from their farm work to come and visit him in the hospital. They plan to help him however they can when he returns home.

Exploring issues with Mr DeGurse

Mr DeGurse and Mr Parker have spent occupational therapy sessions discussing the issues that are important to Mr DeGurse. The biggest hurdle has been for Mr DeGurse to believe that he will indeed be able to return home to his family and his work. Mr DeGurse has many issues that are important to him that he has begun to articulate. He wants to be able to take care of himself totally, so that there is no expectation on his family members to care of him. After accomplishing that goal, he wants to turn his energy back to his farm.

Mr DeGurse and his wife, with their children, have operated the farm with each family member performing particular tasks. It seems to have worked most effectively with each of them having specific roles. This year, Mr DeGurse had started harvesting the corn crop. The crops were harvested for Mr DeGurse by his two sons with generous help from his neighbours. The milk cows are in the barn for the upcoming winter, which will last approximately 4 months in the region in which the family lives.

Mr DeGurse's wife is managing the farm finances. She has always done this task. The children have taken the responsibility for the cows and the other work a family farm requires, even in the winter months. There is much more for them to do than usual, but with some help from already busy neighbours, they seem to be managing.

There is no immediate need for Mr DeGurse's input into the everyday working of the farm at this time. He is already concerned, however, about the numerous spring activities, such as ordering seed, preparing the soil and planting crops.

Mr DeGurse's usual roles on the farm include, but are not exclusively: jointly overseeing the farm's finances with his wife; milking the 30 cows each day using an automatic milking machine in the barn; maintaining and fixing the farm equipment; and operating the tractor to plant and harvest feed for the cows. He wants to be able to return to these activities, if possible, or decide what else he can do on the farm.

Home environment

Mr DeGurse and his family live in a big, two-level farm house. All the bedrooms are on the second floor and there are bathrooms on both floors. The house was built originally by his parents, who now live nearby. It was expanded by the DeGurses over the years.

The barn that houses the cattle and the farm machinery is about 200 m from the house. The barn is reached by a gravel path. The barn for the cows also houses the milking equipment. There is a second building a bit farther from the house that houses all the farm machinery. The machinery is expensive, so Mr DeGurse and his friends have bought some of it cooperatively. The equipment is housed at the DeGurse's farm.

Occupations of Mr DeGurse

Some of Mr DeGurse's occupations have been described already. He and his wife own and operate a large farm on which they keep dairy cows and raise crops such as soybeans and corn. Each member of the family has important responsibilities on the farm.

Mr DeGurse's work occupations also included the day-to-day paperwork and ordering supplies. He was also responsible for monitoring the health of the cows, milking the cows, and supervising the rest of the family members in their activities. He maintained the farm machinery and drove the farm equipment.

Mr and Mrs DeGurse had some leisure time together. They enjoyed going to movies together and having friends over for dinner when their work schedule permitted it. Mr DeGurse also coached a baseball team for teenagers in the summer and was a basketball coach in the winter. The coaching activities included supervising practices in the evenings and coaching at competitive games in a nearby town on some weekend days.

Mr DeGurse is extremely concerned about the farm. There is a lot of work to do. He is uneasy about what he will be able to do on the farm, since he will be using a wheelchair. He is also worried that, even if he is able to do most of his tasks, it will take him too much time to do them and leave him no time to enjoy his family.

Mr DeGurse has explained to Mr Parker that he and his wife are upset that they may not be able to do things together. He is also thinking that he may have to give up all the coaching he has enjoyed for many years. Mr DeGurse has a number of problems to solve with Mr Parker. Consider some of these problems and think about how an understanding of kinematics or movements may help solve some of them.

FUNDAMENTAL CONCEPTS FOR UNDERSTANDING KINEMATICS

There are a number of concepts that are defined here and will be used throughout the chapter. They are terms with specific meanings for biomechanists. These definitions will help you as you work through some of the ideas in the chapter.

- *Kinematics*: Kinematics is the study of movement. It can be described by visual observation, or analysed with various types of measurement equipment. Kinematic measurements describe the motions of objects in space.
- *Distance*: Distance is how far a person or an object moves. For example, a person may be able to reach 40 cm to pick a can off a shelf. The 40 cm is the distance.
- *Displacement*: Displacement is the distance an object travels and it is described using a direction. For example, a person may propel a wheelchair 30 m going north.
- *Speed*: Speed is how quickly an object is going, or is a change in distance with respect to time.
- *Velocity*: Velocity is a change in displacement with respect to time, so it is the same as speed, except it also describes the direction of the speed. For example, a person may be moving at one metre every second (1 m/s), going north.
- *Acceleration*: Acceleration is the change in velocity in a certain time, or with respect to time. Velocity can increase, which is acceleration, or it can decrease, which is deceleration.

MOVEMENT DESCRIPTIONS

Kinematics is the description of the movements we can see or measure. Every time we watch an individual do an occupation, such as climbing up on a tractor, we are watching the kinematics of the movement. We cannot always measure the kinematics in detail, because even something as seemingly simple as climbing up on a tractor is very complex and is difficult to analyse with kinematics.

Kinematic analysis describes a person's movements. These motions are the outcomes of muscular, neurological and learned abilities. Kinematics is not considered to be the science of the forces behind the movements, but really describes the movements themselves.

Kinematic analyses are not restricted to descriptions of human movement. Kinematics has come from the field of mechanics and can also describe movement changes in equipment. The movement of rehabilitation equipment, including wheelchairs or adaptive equipment used to enhance occupations, can be measured using kinematic analysis.

Kinematic movement includes the concepts of displacement, velocity and acceleration. For example, we can measure the distance and direction a person pushes a wheelchair on a gravel path (displacement); the velocity that he or she is able to maintain while manoeuvring on the path; and the acceleration that is needed to get the speed up to what is needed to complete the path. These concepts of movement analysis provide us with some understanding of the expectations required to do an activity.

We can also learn from kinematics information how movements are performed and whether or not different people use the same patterns of movements to do an activity. The advantage of knowing an activity is stereotypical is that we have the opportunity to ask ourselves if particular individuals can approach that pattern of movement. If they may need to change the pattern of movement based on their own physical function, we need to make adaptations. For example, there may be one set of trunk movements required to prepare an automatic milking machine. We need to determine if that set of motions lends itself to adaptations needed by someone who performs movements using a wheelchair.

Displacement, velocity and acceleration can occur in translation. Translation is movement that occurs in a line. Kinematics that are in a specific direction are said to be linear, or to be represented by linear displacement. For example, moving along a straight path can be described using linear kinematics.

The second type of motion is rotation or movement about a set point. Displacement that is about a set point is said to be rotational displacement. Rotation about a set point occurs, for example, when a person bends at the elbow, while pushing a wheelchair up a path.

A third type of motion is general motion, which is translation and rotation working together to produce a movement curve. An example of general motion is a wheelchair user propelling down a path that curves. The person is moving in a linear direction and may also follow the curve of the path by rotating the direction of the wheelchair as the path curves.

Measurements of linear and angular kinematics can be done in a number of ways. Therapists, for example, use goniometers to evaluate the active and passive range of motion (rotational displacement) that individuals use for occupations. This information is used to determine: if the angular kinematics are within normal limits; if they have changed following therapy; or if the amount of rotational movement is adequate for a person to perform occupations.

Kinesiologists can use videotaping, placing markers on a person's joints, and then putting the positions of those markers relative to one another into a computer. The computer programs and output provide the kinesiologist who is analysing movement with information about the rotational and translational kinematics. If this information is collected while someone is engaged in occupations, then the kinesiologist can learn more about movement patterns. The therapist may time movements, for example when the Jebsen Hand Function Test (see Fig. 2.1) is administered. The test requires a person to move objects in specific ways, and the time it takes to carry out the actions is recorded. This is an example of measuring successful displacement. What would be the units of measurement if you could accurately measure the movement path and divide it by the time taken by the person to carry out the movement?

Therapists often consider the displacement, velocity and acceleration of the movement of a person, although they may not think of movements in these specific terms. For the therapist working with an individual such as Mr DeGurse, there are many times during therapy when knowing about kinematics would be helpful. If the therapist knows how much trunk rotation Mr DeGurse has, then occupations can be adapted to accommodate for any reduction in trunk rotation.

Displacement refers to movement that can be straight, change direction, or be curvilinear. Figure 2.2, a person in a wheelchair using a reacher, shows linear displacement at the end of the reacher which is the result of angular displacement (displacement that curves about an axis or point of rotation) at

Figure 2.1 Jebsen Hand Function Test.

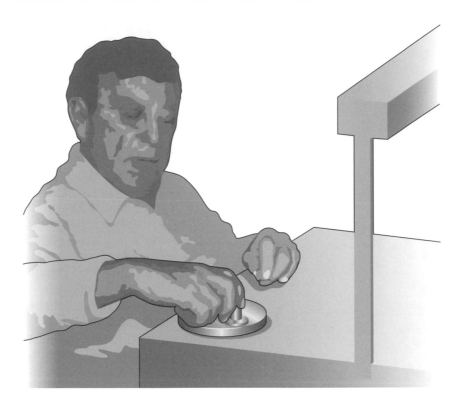

Figure 2.2 Person in a wheelchair using a reacher.

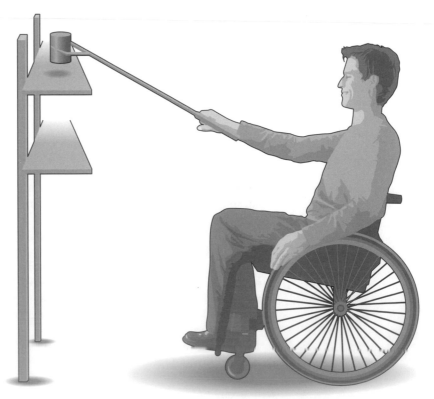

the shoulder and elbow. Another example of an axis of rotation is the centre of the wheel of the wheelchair, where all the spokes converge. The wheel then rotates about this central axis. What would you recommend so that someone with limited angular movement at either of those joints could still reach? Metres are the units of measurement for linear displacement. Degrees or radians are the measurement units for rotational displacement. To be accurate, these measurements include a direction. To consider kinematics to include a direction is useful for a therapist. For example, if the therapist knows that Mr DeGurse must traverse a path through the barn to reach the milking equipment that requires he rotate around other equipment, the therapist needs to know if the wheelchair is designed so that it can follow the curve of the path. If the wheelchair cannot be manoeuvred in the space, accommodations will need to be made.

Joint kinematics

The joint articulating surfaces, between the bones in a person, determine what types of motion can occur at each joint. In some of the carpal bones of the hand, the surfaces of the bones have flat surfaces, so linear motion, or sliding or gliding, occurs between the bones. In other joints, such as the shoulder joint, where the humerus, scapula and clavicle permit a great deal of motion, rotation of the humerus can occur about the centre of the joint and there is a large range of rotation.

Velocity describes how quickly movement occurs. Velocity is in units of metres per second (m/s) with direction. If a joint moves too quickly to allow the ligaments and tendons to move with the joint, the soft structures can tear. For example, if Mr DeGurse swings his legs up onto a tractor too quickly, the soft tissues may be stressed and cause internal damage to his legs.

Acceleration is a change of velocity with respect to time. One can understand the concept of acceleration by thinking of an accelerator on a piece of farm equipment. If the acceleration is increased, the equipment moves more quickly over time. If the acceleration is decreased as the person is bringing the equipment to a stop, then the movement is said to be deceleration. If Mr DeGurse is decelerating a tractor while he is sitting on it, he will need to be careful. Without full trunk muscle function, he may not be able to hold his body in position without constraints of some type. The therapist will have to consider this, if one option for Mr DeGurse is operating the tractor when he returns to farming.

Directions of movement: translation, rotation, general movement

The purpose of this section of the chapter is to further define kinematic principles.

Translation

Translation is movement in a line. Translation can be the result of a number of rotations linked together. Rotation can occur about the shoulder, elbow, wrist and finger joints. The result of all of these rotations occurring simultaneously, or in a sequence, will not be a rotation of the hand necessarily, but can actually be the hand reaching in a straight line (see Fig. 2.2). This translational reach can be lengthened by using a reaching assistive device if necessary. These devices increase the displacement ability of a person and are often used if someone is carrying out occupations when seated.

A person can change the length of distance that is travelled by changing the direction of travel. The Pythagorean theorem explains, mathematically, exactly how much difference in distance there is when moving on a path that requires a turn of 90°, compared to taking a direct path between two points. If a person walks 40 m in one direction, then turns 90° and goes 30 m, the final distance can be determined using the Pythagorean theorem (see Fig. 2.3). Knowing this theorem may be helpful when a therapist is deciding whether or not accommodations may be necessary for a person. For example, if Mr DeGurse needs to go 100 m from the house, and then turn 90° from the first barn to go another 100 m towards the equipment and tractor shed, is it worth considering an alternative route that would go directly from the house to the equipment shed? Knowing how far Mr DeGurse can wheel his chair and working out the distance, the therapist would know if a new path would need to be created or if it were unnecessary.

Rotation is important for functional human movement. Students become familiar with degrees of motion, because they are familiar with rotation at joints and measuring the rotational motion using goniometers. Inadequate

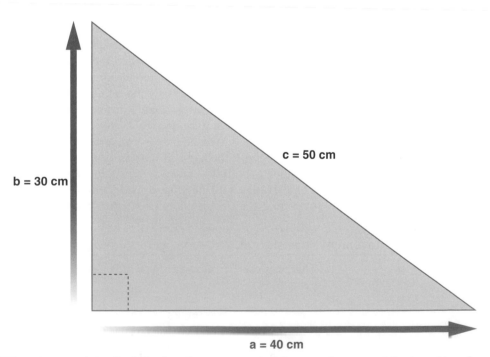

Figure 2.3 The Pythagorean theorem states the following: the square root of the sum of squares of the two sides of a right angle triangle is equal to the hypotenuse (or long side).

range of motion can limit the functional activities an individual is able to perform. Increasing a person's limited range of motion, either through therapy or providing assistive equipment, extends a person's ability to participate in occupations. One example of the necessity of range of motion is that extensive rotation can be required to move levers on some farm equipment. The supplementing of an assistive device could be required to make the device usable by someone who is using a wheelchair.

UNITS OF MEASUREMENT

Units of measurement are the descriptors of numbers used in kinematics. They need to be appropriate and accurate to be meaningful. They also need to be universal numbers. For example, one measurement of weight is a stone, but there are not many populations that would know the meaning of a stone weight.

Measurements are described by numbers, for example '9'. Without a further description of the movement, the number '9' is totally meaningless. To say someone has '2' in the shoulder joint does not provide enough information for anyone to visualise what this means. Does the '2' refer to degrees or radians? Does it imply that the person has a shoulder subluxation that is 2 inches?

Units of measurement are required to complete the description and explanation of a movement, and the standard units of measurement commonly used are described in Table 2.1. These are called SI units (for Système International). Therapists can use the information in the table of units both to describe movements accurately and to understand movement evaluations that are explained in research literature. The units provide information about the measurement. For example, if Mr DeGurse moves at 1 m/s the therapist knows he can move his wheelchair at the same rate as someone else can walk. Knowing Mr DeGurse's velocity in his wheelchair can also provide him and his therapist with information about how long it will take him to move around on his farm.

Table 2.1   Motion and the units of motion.

Motion	International units	Short form of the units
Acceleration	metres per second squared	m/s^2
Angular Acceleration*	degrees per second squared	degrees/s^2
Angular Displacement*	degrees	degrees
Angular Velocity*	degrees per second	degrees/s
Displacement	metres	m
Time	seconds	s
Velocity	metres per second	m/s

*Units of rotation may be measured in radians or degrees, but degrees are commonly used.

DEGREES OF FREEDOM IN MOTION

Degrees of freedom describe all the movements available within a structure or human body. There are three translations. If we think in terms of the human body, these translations can be considered movement along the sagittal, medial–lateral, and frontal planes. There are also three rotations. These three rotations are about the sagittal axis, the medial–lateral axis, and the frontal axis.

Altogether there are six degrees of freedom available: three translations and three rotations. Most joints in the human body cannot achieve movement in all degrees of freedom. For example, the elbow joint, when it is functioning normally, only rotates about the medial–lateral axis, producing flexion and extension. The shoulder joint, because it has a much different structure and is a ball and socket joint, can rotate in all directions. Some of the small joints in the hand, such as the joints between the proximal phalanges and the metacarpals, can rotate, but also have a small amount of glide. The number of degrees of freedom available at a joint is the total of all the movements at the joint and is related to the structure of the joint. The more degrees of freedom a joint has, usually the more mobile it is.

These movements may be altered if a person has experienced a disease process. The range of motion at joints may become reduced. For example, if a person has paralysis of some of the trunk musculature and the lower limbs, there is decreased voluntary range of motion of the trunk. If the spinal cord injury is complete, as is the case for Mr DeGurse, then there is no voluntary range of motion in the legs at all. This decreased range of motion of the trunk and lack of control in the legs, results in occupational performances which will need to be adapted or discontinued.

The body, as a whole, can also exhibit up to the total of six degrees of freedom. For example, if Mr DeGurse practises rolling from side to side on a therapy plinth in preparation for lower extremity dressing, he is rolling about the longitudinal axis. If he reaches down to his feet, he is rotating his trunk about the medial–lateral axis. A therapist working with Mr DeGurse will want to consider the translations and rotations that he has available to him.

UNDERSTANDING HOW PEOPLE MOVE

We may help the people we work with more effectively if we understand how they move. For example, a therapist may work with someone with paraplegia who has retained hand and arm movement, but has limited trunk movement. The therapist may help the individual perform activities, by extending the arm reach or total distance the person can reach from a wheelchair with a reacher, and generally accomplish the skills in which they wish to be engaged. The therapist and individual may need to determine how to modify the environment to enhance productivity at work. The individual will benefit from the therapist understanding how movement is measured and the implications of the movement limitations.

QUALITY OF MOVEMENT

An occupational therapy student can visually examine how an occupation is done by an individual. An experienced observer is someone who observes the quality of a movement more accurately than someone who is beginning to observe movement patterns. Some of the components of movement quality include speed, smoothness, and accuracy of the movement. The quality of a person's movements can be altered or reduced when an injury or a disease occurs. Parkinson's disease, for example, interferes with an individual's ability to move adequately and hence interferes with activities that a person would like to perform. Performance of movements may be slowed and the person may be unable to initiate movement. Researchers,[1] however, suggest that when people who have Parkinson's disease can do reach-to-grasp actions with their upper extremities, they can perform them in a functional and coordinated manner.

Different functional abilities are evident, even among people who have the same disability. Therapists, through experience, learn to see these functional abilities and help the person to perform occupations. One way that therapists can observe the quality of movement is to videotape and replay the movement.

FUNDAMENTALS OF VIDEO RECORDING AND ANALYSIS FOR OCCUPATIONAL THERAPY APPLICATIONS

(Content for this section provided by Dr DI Miller, with permission.)

A technique that helps therapists to analyse movement is to record the movement with a video camera and replay the activity. Therapists can apply video recording to document an individual's temporal and motor performance, including initial, intermediate and final assessments. Therapists can provide in-service training for therapists and assistants, for example recording patient transfers and therapists' teaching methods. Video recording can enhance the analysis of particular motor skills; provide feedback for individuals of their performance during a session; indicate evidence of effective treatment methods over time; and document occupational performance for insurance purposes.

Video recording has advantages over many of the measurement systems that can be used to analyse movement. It is relatively inexpensive and camcorders are usually available from institutional or personal sources. Camcorders can be easily set up to capture the desired field of view and can be left to simply run, so an extra person is not required to operate the camera. The system is portable and can be used in a clinical, work or home setting.

Ethics and confidentiality are involved when using a video system. The student or therapist must inform individuals or co-workers that they are being videotaped and explain the purpose of the videotaping session. Therapists should only use videos for presentations with the express written consent of the individuals on the tape. Also, videotapes must be kept in a secure location as they are part of an individual's confidential record. It is a good idea to have a separate videotape for each individual to keep in the record and also for ease of organisation if serial monitoring is being done.

Planning and setting up video recording

If possible, those being videotaped should wear clothing that allows joint and limb motion to be clearly seen, for example short sleeve shirts and shorts that are not too loose. It is easiest to see action if the background is unobstructed. There should be good contrast between the subject and the background.

The student or clinician should determine the best camera position to record the action. The most secure position for the camcorder is to have it on a tripod in a place that does not obstruct normal traffic patterns. One should document the camera protocol so that the camera setup can be the same if an individual is videotaped in a series of sessions for assessment or treatment.

It is best to position the camera as far away from the subject as possible, and then zoom in to capture the desired field of view, and to have as large an image as possible. There should be a vertical and/or a horizontal reference in the background, and an object of known length in the plane of action. This object can be placed in the field of view before or after videotaping the individual. Another option is to measure the dimensions of a reference object, such as a chair or desk that is in the plane of action. The camera should be level from front to back and side to side. To focus, zoom in as far as possible, then focus, then zoom back out to the desired field size.

The date and time should be recorded on the videotape. The therapist can superimpose 'date/time' information on the videotape as long as it does not obstruct the motion to be analysed. As an alternative if this information obscures the view of the individual, date/time information can be put in at the beginning and the end of a session. The date/time should be synchronised before each data collection begins. A digital watch can be used as a common source for the time synchronisation.

Set the shutter speed according to the light that is available. The shutter may work at 1/125th, 1/150th, 1/500th, or 1/1000th, or in some cases, even faster. The less light that is available, the slower the shutter will have to be to see the motion on the videotape. The faster the action, the faster the shutter will have to be to eliminate blur. Generally an exposure of 1/30th of a second (no shutter) will result in a blurry picture and will not be clear enough for clinical purposes. Set the shutter speed to at least 1/100th of a second, otherwise single freeze frames viewed in a frame-by-frame advance mode will likely be blurry.

Run the camera with an alternating current (AC) power cord, if possible, rather than on a battery. If battery operation is the only option, be sure that the battery is well-charged and that a spare, charged battery is available. If transporting the equipment in cold weather conditions, be sure that the battery is not left in the cold and that all the equipment and videotapes are warmed up before use.

Videotaping locomotion

The camera should be secured to a tripod which is level and stationary during the videotaping. While it is customary to record locomotion from the side, views from the front and/or the back will also provide useful information. Marks should be placed at regular intervals along the side of the walkway (for example at 100 cm or 1 m intervals) so step length can be estimated. The National Television Standards Committee (NTSC) video recording frame rate (standard for North America, Central America, Japan, parts of South America and the South Pacific) is 29.97 frames per second (fps); the Phase Alternation Line (PAL, standard for UK, Germany, the Netherlands) and the Séquential Couleur avec Mémoire (SECAM, standard for France, eastern Europe and the Middle East) frame rates are 25 fps. By counting the frames, support (when the foot is on the ground) and swing times (when the foot is swinging forward for the next contact with the ground) can be determined. For individuals with mobility problems, the time to cover a given distance may simply be determined by using the time information displayed on the screen.

Videotaping fundamentals to ensure useful images are acquired

It is a good idea to have a separate videotape for each individual if a series of assessments is being made. The individual tapes can be kept in the individual's file and confidentiality can be ensured. Comments recorded by the therapist or individual on the audio portion of the tape may be useful but be careful, because anything that is said while the tape is running will be recorded.

Be sure that either a blank videotape is in the camera or that you are past the point of existing data that you want to keep, when you begin recording. Turn the camera power 'on'. Remove the lens cap and look through the viewer to establish the field of view by zooming in and out. To focus the camera, have someone stand in the centre of the field of view. A reference object could also be used for this purpose. Set the focus to 'manual', because you can control the focus. Automatic focus will change the focus so that whatever is in the centre of the view is in focus. Once the focus is set to manual, zoom in as close as possible to the centre of the field, which represents a maximum image and minimum depth of field. Adjust the focus. Once a sharp focus has been achieved, zoom out to encompass the field in which the action is to take place, but try to have the image of your subject as large as possible.

Always let the camcorder run continuously for at least a minute at the beginning of the tape. This needs to be done once, usually at the beginning of the tape. Recording this blank tape will permit the videotapes to be digitised using a computerised video digitising system, if that is to be used at a later time. Otherwise, the digitising system will not have sufficient tape with which to begin the time encoding which must precede any analyses.

Start the camera well before the person enters the field of view or before the designated action is to begin. Allow the camera to run beyond the end of the action as it will rewind slightly when the recording stops. Videotape is relatively inexpensive, so use more rather than less.

Finally, keep careful records at the time you collect the information. This information should include the camera height, distance to the subject, focal length, lens distance setting, and information about your individual, including the person's age, height, weight, skill background, movement difficulties and any other information that might be needed when reviewing or using the tapes at a later time.

Figure 2.4   Video clip: person rising from a chair.

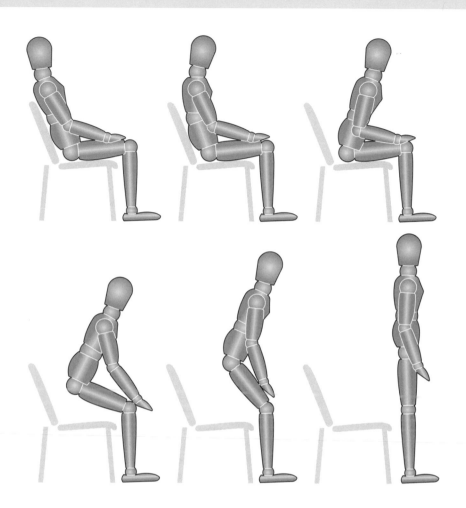

Videotaping is not used frequently during treatment sessions, but it provides a valuable tool for observing movement information and a lasting record for the therapist. A student or therapist can try to evaluate the technique's utility in the practice environment of the person. Figure 2.4 shows pictures clipped from a videotape. The clips show the movements involved in going from sitting to standing. What activities would you videotape in a clinic? How could you use video clips?

ADVANCED INFORMATION ABOUT KINEMATICS: STUDIES EVALUATING OCCUPATIONS AND KINEMATICS

Some movements that are relevant to occupational therapists have been scientifically analysed, to determine their kinematic features. Specific movements that have been evaluated include wheelchair propulsion, reaching and grasping, moving from sitting to standing, climbing stairs, and the interaction between head and scapular positions. Some of the study results will be examined here to demonstrate the use of kinematics in understanding movement in individuals who may have difficulty moving, or who use assistive devices and technology to move.

Researchers do not always evaluate just one aspect of kinematics, such as the angular movements at one joint. They often work to identify and understand many movement parameters that may contribute to a specific task. For example, Bednarczyk & Sanderson[2] evaluated wheelchair propulsion in children and adults with spinal cord injuries. These researchers found that the velocity of the adults was greater (2.4 m/s) than the propulsion velocity of the children (2.3 m/s). Both groups spent approximately 24% of the wheel cycle in propulsion. The authors suggested that studies of adult wheelchair users might apply to paediatric populations for the movement parameter of percentage of the wheelchair propulsion spent in grasp.

Elbow kinematics have been found to differ between pushing a wheelchair with a shorter arc of the hand in contact with the rim, and when using a movement that has the hand pushing on the rim through more of the arc of the wheel rim.[3] Wheelchair racing techniques have also been evaluated. Athletes who race wheelchairs push faster as they increase speed,[4] but they do not change the angle of the push on the wheelchair.[5]

Reaching and grasping are basic movement patterns that are required for many tasks. Adding purpose to these activities, rather than simulating a purpose, or performing the movement without purpose, may affect the performance of the activity in a positive manner. This finding has been determined through evaluating the kinematics of the movement. Researchers[6] evaluated a reaching activity and an activity that did not have a noticeable reason for its performance. The researchers found that when people performed purposeful reach, they demonstrated shorter movement times and higher peak velocities than they did when executing an impoverished activity. This finding supported the tenet that goal-directed activities might enhance movement performance. The results of this study imply that students should work with people to determine movements that are meaningful to the individuals, because finding purposeful movement may encourage improved movement patterns.

Structuring upper extremity tasks to include occupational relevance, sometimes called embeddedness, appears to change the parameters of the movement. Natural context may facilitate the outcome of motor learning in individuals who do not have disabilities.[7] Reaching motions are organised depending on the task requirements.[8] Embedded purpose may also enhance the movement patterns of individuals who have neurological impairment. Comparing a task of scooping coins off a table with simulating the task demonstrated that the presence of the object facilitated improved movement in individuals with neurological impairment.[9]

Grasping activities can demonstrate differences between individuals who do not have movement difficulties and those people who do have problems. The better these differences are understood, the more readily improvement of movements or recommended equipment or environmental changes may occur. Research that evaluated grasping activities in children with cerebral palsy and those who developed without cerebral palsy determined that movements are often exaggerated in children with cerebral palsy. These children often do not possess control mechanisms to anticipate how widely they should open their hands for different-sized objects.[10]

Individuals with Huntington's disease with chorea differed from people without the disease when performing a reaching movement.[11] Individuals with the disease had hand path movements that were not straight, but had initial velocities that were similar to individuals without the disease. The authors suggested that the presence of sub-movements in people with Huntington's disease might be an adaptive strategy to improve accuracy, or a deficit in controlling deceleration.

Reaching for an object results in kinematic or spatial difficulties for individuals who have experienced left brain injuries.[12] Hermsdorfer et al suggested that people who have experienced left brain damage use different strategies for reaching an object. Arm movements in a reaching task in individuals who have sustained a stroke indicate that the movements are different than in individuals who have not sustained a stroke. The movements took longer, were more segmented, had larger movement errors, and were more variable. These individuals also tended to move their trunk during the reach, but only if the deficit was large.[13]

Movement patterns in the upper extremity in individuals who have experienced a cerebral vascular accident appear smoother and more efficient when the task has a real goal compared with when the activity is simulated.[9] It appears, as would be expected, that having a neurological condition may interfere with reaching and grasping. There is support for the idea that ensuring that the movement has purpose will improve the kinematic parameters of the movement.

Reach may be affected by scapular rotation. Head position, in turn, may affect scapular rotation[14] and scapular elevation.[15] Increase in head flexion in the sagittal plane occurs with an increase in scapular angle. As the humerus elevates, the scapula upwardly rotates, changing the inferior angle.[14] Scapular loading indicates that light loads increase the scapulo-humeral rhythm from approximately 3:1 to 4:1, but that heavier loads increase this relationship from approximately 2:1 to 5:1 with arm elevation. If the humerus range of motion is passive, the rhythm between the scapula and the humerus decreases from 8:1 to 2:1. These results suggest that the simple linear 2:1 scapula to humeral movement ratio may be oversimplified and that therapists may expect these ratios to vary with load and humeral movement.[16]

Other kinematic difficulties may result from a neurological or orthopaedic problem. Elbow kinematic patterns are similar in people who have rheumatoid arthritis, but the angle of the elbow that a person actually used was 15–20° less than was available to that individual. This suggests there is a need for a residual range of motion.[17]

Another example of occupational difficulty following decreased range of motion is that adequate rotation is required in the lower extremity joints to assure safe stair climbing.[18] Lower limb angular displacements are influenced by the dimensions of the stairs during stair climbing. The knee flexion angle can vary, depending on the staircase, suggesting that the dimensions of the stairs influence the kinematics of the lower limb.[19]

SUMMARY

Therapists can benefit from the information they acquire about kinematic variables. This information will help them understand the movements their individuals make. Therapists can measure the time, and many other kinematic variables, that constitute the physical components of an activity. Therapists who measure kinematics have sound knowledge about whether or not a person is doing the activity at a speed that is functional for the occupations the person wishes to perform.

Therapists should also apply the concepts of kinematics when they determine therapy plans. For example, they can determine if velocity or acceleration need to be changed on powered mobility equipment, or if augmentative communication devices will make the equipment more useful for individuals. Therapists will enhance their decisions about treatment techniques by considering the movements required for an activity in terms of the kinematic requirements of the activity and the movement patterns and functions available to the individuals they work with.

Readers who have completed this chapter will now be able to read the literature that addresses the kinematic issues of people with physical problems. They will be able to use that knowledge to improve their therapy and assist the people they work with.

QUESTIONS BASED ON THE CASE

1. What will be the major issues of mobility for Mr DeGurse? Draw out the DeGurse farm buildings on a piece of paper, as they are described. Can you design routes so that he will not have to move long distances? He will have difficulties with his home layout, because he is using a wheelchair. Do you know the dimensions of a standard wheelchair? Can you determine the space needed for the wheelchair to be rotated 360°?

2. What activities might be hampered by his limitation in how far his arms can reach because he will be undertaking all his activities sitting down? When you are considering these activities, you should think of the broad range of occupations that he wants to engage in. Can he carry out his own self care? Can he work in the barn? Can he use farm machinery? If you are not familiar with farms, can you find someone who does know about them? Purdue University in West Lafayette, Indiana, USA is one university that has a group of people working on farm equipment for disabilities. Can you find the website on the internet for this group? Are there other websites that you can find that would be useful for Mr DeGurse? Providing him with information will alleviate some of his concerns about his abilities to work on his farm.

3. Mr Parker and Mr DeGurse together can figure out how to adapt his work so that he can milk the cows and drive the tractor with hand controls. The speed at which he can get to his activities, however, has slowed because he has to push his wheelchair over surfaces such as gravel and grass. What advice, based on the literature described in this chapter, could you give him about wheelchair propulsion techniques, so that he can increase his propelling velocity? The environmental factors that influence people who have movement problems have not been discussed in detail in this book yet, but can you think of how the ground characteristics on Mr DeGurse's farm are going to hamper his ability to use his wheelchair?

continued overpage

4. If the path from the house to the barn is downhill and he starts moving at 2 m/s and ends up at the barn travelling at 5.5 m/s, what is his average acceleration? Can you think of a way that he might slow himself down safely when he reaches the barn?

5. Mr DeGurse must manoeuvre his wheelchair around the large barn. He has to go 60 m in one direction to get to the end of the barn, then turn at a right angle (90°) and go 80 m to get to the milking equipment. To save time and his energy, he and the therapist are considering putting a concrete path from the front of the barn directly to the milking machine. How much distance will this save him? Do you think it is worth the effort and expense to make this change? There is often a trade-off between improved function and cost. Sometimes it is worth the cost to make the change. Other times, increasing a person's strength, changing movement patterns or adapting the occupation can be used instead. Do you think that there are other ways that this problem can be solved?

Laboratory Exercise: Examples of Kinematics Applied to Improve Occupational Performance

1. A wheelchair user propels herself over a straight path that is 100 m long in 150 s. What was her average velocity and what are the units of velocity?

2. A person pushing a wheelchair changes speed from 2 m/s to 3 m/s in 2 seconds. What is his average acceleration during that time?

3. Do the following activity yourself. Reach for a can of soup from a kitchen cupboard, take the can off the shelf, and put it on the counter.
   a. What was the displacement of the can?
   b. Now, do the same activity sitting down facing the shelf (preferably using a wheelchair if you have one available). What is the displacement in this situation? Is there greater or less displacement when you do the activity sitting down compared to when you do it standing up?
   c. Repeat the activity a third time with the chair sideways to the shelf.
   d. Repeat the activities described from a to c, only this time use a reacher. Is there a difference in the total displacement of the can?
   e. If one of the techniques allows your hand to have more displacement than another technique when you are in the seated position, why do you think that occurs?

4. Complete the activities again, trying to go as quickly as possible and using a stopwatch to measure your time. What are the differences in the velocities using the different positions? What are the differences when using a reacher and not using a reacher? Can you describe the changes that you made to increase the velocity of the movement? If you have videotaped the action, can you see the differences more clearly? If you targeted a certain spot on the counter to place the can, was there any difference in your accuracy at different speeds?

5. If you have access to a video camera, do the activities in questions 3 and 4 again with a video position in the front, so you can get a view of the frontal plane. Next, videotape the activities from the side so you get a sagittal view. Review the videotapes as described in the section in the text. You should be able to perceive more details of the activities.

6. Try another occupational performance task and complete the above exercise.

7. Pick an activity or part of an activity that you do for leisure. During that activity, can you determine the range of motion (ROM) that you used in your shoulder? Would you describe the movement as linear or angular? How would you describe the movement at your elbow and your wrist?

REFERENCES

1. Castiello U, Bennett KM. The bilateral reach-to-grasp movement of Parkinson's disease subjects. Brain 1997; 120(Pt 4):593–604.
2. Bednarczyk JH, Sanderson DJ. Kinematics of wheelchair propulsion in adults and children with spinal cord injury. Arch Phys Med Rehabil 1994; 75(12):1327–1334.
3. Rudins A, Laskowski ER, Growney ES, Cahalan TD, An KN. Kinematics of the elbow during wheelchair propulsion: a comparison of two wheelchairs and two stroking techniques. Arch Phys Med Rehabil 1997; 78(11):1204–1210.
4. Wang YT, Deutsch H, Morse M, Hedrick B, Millikan T. Three-dimensional kinematics of wheelchair propulsion across racing speeds. Adapt Phys Activity Q 1995; 12(1): 78–89.
5. Goosey VL, Fowler NE, Campbell IG. A kinematic analysis of wheelchair propulsion techniques in senior male, senior female, and junior male athletes. Adapt Phys Activity Q 1997; 14(2):156–165.
6. Lin KC, Wu CY, Trombly CA. Effects of task goal on movement kinematics and line bisection performance in adults without disabilities. Am J Occup Ther 1998; 52(3): 179–187.
7. Ma HI, Trombly CA, Robinson-Podolski C. The effect of context on skill acquisition and transfer. Am J Occup Ther 1999; 53(2):138–144.
8. van Vliet P. An investigation of the task specificity of reaching: implications for retraining. Physiother Theory Pract 1993; 9(2):69–76.
9. Wu C, Trombly CA, Lin K, Tickle-Degnen L. Effects of object affordances on reaching performance in persons with and without cerebrovascular accident. Am J Occup Ther 1998; 52(6):447–456.
10. Cope SM, Trombly CA. Grasping in children with and without cerebral palsy: a kinematic analysis. Scand J Occup Ther 1998; 5(2):59–68.
11. Quinn L, Hamel V, Flanagan JR, Kaminski T, Rubin A. Control of multijoint arm movements in Huntington's disease. J Neurol Rehabil 1997; 11(1):47–60.
12. Hermsdorfer J, Mai N, Spatt J, Marquardt C, Velkamp R. Kinematic analysis of movement imitation in apraxia. Brain 1996; 119(Pt 5):1575–1586.
13. Cirstea MC, Levin MF. Compensatory strategies for reaching in stroke. Brain 2000; 123(Pt 5):940–953.
14. Ludewig PM, Cook TM. The effect of head position on scapular orientation and muscle activity during shoulder elevation. J Occup Rehabil 1996; 6(3):147–158.
15. Ludewig PM, Cook TM, Nawoczenski DA. Three-dimensional scapular orientation and muscle activity at selected positions of humeral elevation. J Orthop Sports Phys Ther 1996; 24(2):57–65.

16. McQuade KJ, Smidt GL. Dynamic scapulohumeral rhythm: the effects of external resistance during elevation of the arm in the scapular plane. J Orthop Sports Phys Ther 1998; 27(2):125–133.

17. Packer TL, Wyss UP, Costigan P. Elbow kinematics during sit-to-stand-to-sit of subjects with rheumatoid arthritis. Arch Phys Med Rehabil 1994; 75(8):900–907.

18. Asplund DJ, Hall SJ. Kinematics and myoelectric activity during stair-climbing ergometry. J Orthop Sports Phys Ther 1995; 22(6):247–253.

19. Livingston LA, Stevenson JM, Olney SJ. Stairclimbing kinematics on stairs of differing dimensions. Arch Phys Med Rehabil 1991; 72(6):398–402.

Chapter 3

Kinetics: the implications of adding force during occupations

Kinetics is the study of human movement that involves both the movements and the forces that produce the movements. So the difference between understanding kinematics (as discussed in the previous chapter) and kinetics, is that when thinking about and studying kinetics, the therapist learns about the forces creating the movements as well as all the forces acting on the body, both internally and externally, as opposed to learning about the movements themselves.

The forces on the body are exerted internally by muscles. Therapists work to strengthen muscles for movement, or to help a person when muscles do not work well because of a disease process or injury. Forces are also exerted from outside the body. The environment, the therapist, or adaptive equipment such as a wheelchair,[1] prosthesis,[2] or orthoses[3-6] may exert an external force on a person. It is important for us to know what forces are and how they work. There are a number of characteristics that will be explained in this chapter, including the definition of forces. The concepts of torque and levers will be explained in a manner that enables therapists to use these concepts in their work.

The following case study describes someone who can benefit from a therapist's understanding of kinetics. Keep this individual in mind as you work through the chapter, then answer the questions at the end of the chapter related to this person.

CASE STUDY: MS JOSEPHINE TASKER

Ms Josephine Tasker is a 63-year-old individual who lives in a rural community that is isolated and about 400 km from the closest town. She has lived in the community all her life. She lives alone but, since most of the people in the community of 300 people have always been there as well, she knows them all.

Ms Tasker has had Type II diabetes for about 20 years. About a year ago, she had a seriously infected foot because of the side-effects of diabetes. She was taken to a hospital in the town 400 km away. There she had her right leg amputated above the knee. She was fitted with a prosthesis and sent home with a walker and a manual wheelchair. Sometimes she has skin breakdown on her leg in the area of the prosthesis and uses the wheelchair until her skin heals.

Ms Tasker lives on social assistance. The amount of money that she receives is enough for her to maintain her two room home and to buy food with a little left over to replace her clothing when it wears out.

The setting

The setting is Ms Tasker's home and the rural community in which she lives. Her two room home consists of a main area for cooking and sitting and a smaller room that she uses as a bedroom. She does not have running water or electricity. She uses a woodstove for heating and for cooking. She gets her water from the community well. She has an outhouse that she uses as a toilet.

The house is situated on the only street in the village. The village road outside her home is a dirt road. The village is on a small lake.

The community is isolated, being about 3 hours from the closest town. It is accessible only by a dirt road. The village has a small store for purchasing food and some basic necessities. Because of its location, it is not possible to grow any food in the surrounding area and all provisions must be brought in from other locations. There are a number of people in the community who have substance abuse problems and these would not be people whom Ms Tasker could count on to help her out, but some of the people in her age group are helpful. She has someone who can bring her wood and water when she needs it, but otherwise she is essentially self-sufficient and quietly independent.

The occupational therapist

The occupational therapist is Marjorie Stauffer who graduated from an occupational therapy programme one year ago. She was not familiar with the area of the country where she works until she started her position there after she graduated. She can communicate with other therapists about individuals, but she does most of her work alone. She is either flown in to the small communities by float plane or drives. She is part of a publicly funded group of therapists who do rural practice.

The area that she is responsible for in the practice is about 600 square kilometres. She is responsible for any occupational therapy that is done in the area. This means she works with people of all ages who have various difficulties. She finds the work challenging and must be very creative in her solutions to help those she works with because most of them live in small villages with minimal access to healthcare services.

The individual

Ms Tasker is a woman who has spent her life in the small community in which she lives. Her family has been there for many generations. She was married, but her husband died 20 years ago while he was out hunting for food. She has no children. She is a person who is used to making do with few material possessions and is used to hardship at times.

She has been aware for some time that she might have difficulty because of her diabetes. A number of people in her community have the same problem and she has watched the progression of the disease in them.

She knows she will always have difficulty walking and that infections and skin problems will always be things that could happen to her again. It is difficult for her to maintain a level of cleanliness for herself and her house that would make it less likely that she would have many infections. She knows life is going to be more difficult than it previously has been. It will be harder for her to get around. It may be impossible for her to maintain her independence, but she is not sure where else she could live or how she could make things easier. She is getting a bit more money from the government, because she is now labelled as disabled. This money will help her somewhat, but there are still many problems to overcome.

Physical abilities

Ms Tasker has many problems with her physical abilities. She is unable to ambulate any long distances with her prosthesis and her walker because she fatigues through being very overweight. The ground surfaces around her house are uneven and hard to walk on, especially after it has been raining. She finds it difficult to get around with the wheelchair, because of the ground. She had to get hard tyres on her wheelchair, because it would have been very difficult to have punctures fixed, so it is difficult to manoeuvre.

Ms Tasker has full use of her arms, but because of the diabetes, her weight problem and her fatigue, she finds it is difficult to do many things for herself. She finds carrying things hard, and even taking care of herself is awkward.

Another problem she is starting to have because of the diabetes is poor vision. This has been an issue for a couple of years. The glasses she was prescribed around the same time she was at the hospital for her surgery seem to be helping.

Emotional status

Ms Tasker is quite accepting of her physical abilities and limitations. She is not particularly upset by having had the amputation or by the diabetes. She seems to take the problems as just things that happen in life and is accepting of them.

Ms Tasker does not feel totally isolated by the restrictions created by her diabetes. Her friends come to visit and she enjoys spending time having coffee and talking with them. They sometimes play cards.

Exploring issues with Ms Tasker

Marjorie Stauffer is visiting Ms Tasker's community for 3 days to work with Ms Tasker, some children who have fetal alcohol syndrome and their families, and two other members of the community who also have complications due to diabetes.

Ms Stauffer and Ms Tasker discuss some of the issues that Ms Tasker has. Ms Stauffer is concerned about Ms Tasker's ability to maintain her self-care and look after her diabetic condition. They are both aware that if Ms Tasker does not establish a method to maintain cleanliness, do her self-care, and perform her chores, including cooking and keeping her woodstove fire working, she will have major problems living alone and avoiding further complications from the diabetes.

Ms Tasker is very concerned about her general lack of strength. Without strong arm muscles she finds that doing the occupations that enable her to survive are becoming increasingly arduous. She finds it difficult to do everything, from opening the heavy wooden door of her home to lifting the wood from the floor into her stove. She finds it challenging to make meals standing at her counter. She finds getting from place to place difficult and even harder when the weather is rainy or cold. She is not sure if the weakness she feels is a result of the diabetes or from the time she spent in the hospital and was not active. Whatever the reason, the inability to do almost anything without a huge effort is limiting to her. She does not know how much help she can get from her friends because they are close to the same age she is and they also have physical problems of their own.

The community consists of people who all belong to the same group of indigenous people and who work to help one another when possible. The elders of the community, consisting of 5 of the older men and women of the group, are concerned about Ms Tasker, but do not know how it would be possible to help her with the limited resources of other members of the group.

Occupations of Ms Tasker

Ms Tasker lives a simple life. She has always been able to meet her needs to survive and to enjoy the community suppers or meetings with her friends. Her occupations have always been fairly limited, because she does not need much and she does not have money to purchase many things, even if she did need them.

She does need to take care of herself, including maintaining cleanliness and controlling her diabetes. At present she needs to work around her home. Although it is small, it is very difficult for her to use a wheelchair because the work surfaces are at a height for a standing person.

Ms Tasker would also like to maintain her relationships with her friends and participate in the community meals and ceremonies that are happening. She has always been involved in doing the beadwork for the formal clothing worn for community ceremonies.

The community has difficulty maintaining unity, because many of the younger people either have substance abuse problems or have moved to larger places. People like Ms Tasker are needed to keep up the traditions of the community. Although Ms Tasker is very independent, she is of an age within the group that she understands the need for maintaining some of the traditions. Her participation in the community has always been paramount for her own wellbeing. Consider some of the issues that have been described. Ms Tasker has a simple lifestyle, but imagine the complexity that has been introduced because she is living with the problems associated with having diabetes and using a lower extremity prosthesis. Both of these physical changes introduce problems into every aspect of her life. You should be able to think of a number of solutions for some of the problems mentioned here as you read through the information about kinetics described in this chapter.

FUNDAMENTAL CONCEPTS FOR UNDERSTANDING KINETICS

There are many concepts that will be used in this chapter that are important to understand.

- *Anthropometry*: Anthropometry is the study of the dimensions or size of a person. This study includes measurements of the whole person or of segments, such as the length of a finger.
- *Force*: A force is the product of mass and acceleration (F = ma). Forces cause movements, stop movements, or change the direction of movements. Forces can also help a person maintain standing or sitting stability and balance.
- *Mass*: Mass is the amount of matter contained in an object. Mass is often related to weight, because the force of gravity affects the mass of objects on earth.
- *Mechanical advantage*: Mechanical advantage is a quantitative (or numeric) measure of the mechanical effectiveness of a lever or other device, e.g. a pulley. The ratio of the length of the force arm to the length of the resistance arm for a given lever is that lever's mechanical advantage.
- *Moment of force*: Moment of force is the quantity of force times the distance between the force and its application.
- *Momentum*: Momentum is mass times velocity.
- *Strength*: Strength is the amount of force a person or a muscle can exert.
- *Weight*: Weight is mass times the force of gravity, or the pull towards the centre of the earth.

UNITS OF MEASUREMENT

There are many measurements that are used when discussing kinetics, as there are when describing kinematics. Each of these measurements has a unit associated with it. Measurements are given in either British or International units. Since most countries use the International (or SI) units as their standard, they will be the usual units described here.

- *Force:* The units of force are kilograms times metres per second squared ($kg \cdot m/s^2$), and are known as Newtons (N). A force is thought of as having a point of application, a magnitude or size and a direction.
- *Mass:* Mass is measured in kilograms (kg).
- *Moment of force:* A moment of force is measured in $kg \cdot m^2/s^2$, or Newton·metres (N·m).
- *Momentum:* Momentum is the mass times velocity, so the units of momentum will be $kg \cdot m/s$.
- *Weight:* In British Thermal units, weight is measured in pounds. In SI units, weight is mass in kilograms times the force of gravity in m/s^2, or Newtons (N). When we weigh ourselves, we actually should be recording our weight in Newtons, rather than kilograms. Kilograms represent mass rather than weight. To determine our weight in Newtons, we must multiply our mass in kilograms by $9.81 \, m/s^2$. $9.81 \, m/s^2$ is the acceleration due to gravity that pulls us down towards the earth. If you think about it, multiplying our weight by such a large number would definitely make us seem like we weigh a lot more.

ANTHROPOMETRY: A PERSON'S BODY DIMENSIONS

Anthropometry is the study of the dimensions of the human body. The averages of lengths of the trunk, arms and legs are important because they are needed to understand how a person can fit into environmental characteristics or have difficulties in relationship to the environment. Environmental characteristics include everything from the size of a chair to the dimensions of airplane cockpit controls.

Average weights are needed to determine the design of furniture, devices and equipment. They are needed to determine how sturdy furniture needs to be and how strong lifts must be to move a wheelchair and a person from one floor of a residence to a higher or lower level.

Average heights, limb lengths, weights and other physical dimensions vary between genders and among ethnic groups. Averaging information has limited use, at times, within the occupational therapy context. The specific limb lengths, torso height and other measurements of a person are essential when a therapist is ordering a custom-built wheelchair for that individual. For example, the therapist cannot provide Ms Tasker, who has diabetes and an amputation, with a wheelchair for the 'average' sized person, because Ms Tasker will have less weight in her lower extremities than she would before she had her prosthesis fitted. In addition, the prosthesis weighs less than a limb, so Ms Tasker's centre of gravity will have moved backwards when she is sitting down. She also has more potential for falling backwards unless some adaptations are made to her wheelchair. The potential for pressure sores, the inability to push a manual chair or drive a power chair, and a mismatch between the wheelchair and the person's furniture, such as a desk or dining room table, can all be minimized if correct measuring is done by the therapist. If Ms Tasker were to have a pressure sore on her buttocks in the wheelchair, she would have more difficulty healing than would someone without diabetes. Therefore her seating requirements will be a high priority. The success of wheelchair use is related to the fit among the person, the wheelchair and the person's environment. The therapist working with Ms Tasker will need to be creative in helping her adapt to her environment, or will have to consider methods of altering her environment.

MOMENTUM: MAKING CLINICAL USE OF MASS AND VELOCITY

Momentum is the term used when the mass of an object, or person, is multiplied by the velocity at which the mass is moving. If a heavy person is sitting in a heavy wheelchair and is being pushed down a hill, the momentum will be greater than if the person and/or the wheelchair were lighter in weight. The wheelchair may be difficult to stop, particularly if either the person is heavy or the wheelchair is moving quickly. The person and wheelchair will continue moving down the hill unless acted on by a strong enough force that is working opposite to the movement in order to stop it.

Therapists can incorporate momentum into their teaching. For example, if people need to move from a chair to a bed, they can position themselves so that by increasing their velocity, they can move their own mass. Ms Tasker will find it difficult to manoeuvre, but it will be easier if she can consider using momentum to move herself around. The problems she will need to deal with in terms of momentum include the need to move heavy objects, such as wood for her stove. The mass of the wood will be great, and it will be difficult to start it moving, but once it is going, it may be difficult for her to decelerate it. Momentum must be considered when the therapist and Ms Tasker work together to organise her environment to meet her needs.

FORCE

The concept of force is fundamental for understanding kinetics. Force is also one of the attributes or requirements of most occupations and underlies movement and kinematics. The option of having no force requirements for working equipment is difficult to obtain. Muscles must exert some force in order even to move the weight of a body component, in order to be effective. Occupational therapists measure force routinely during clinical work. An understanding of force also provides occupational therapists with important research information.[7]

Many different movements have been evaluated using kinetic measures and changes in kinetic variables. The information gleaned from this research can benefit occupational therapists when working with people who have physical disabilities. Evaluation and documentation of forces for specific populations would help occupational therapists determine an optimum force output and relate that output to occupations. Ms Tasker has reduced strength or force output compared with what she had previously. This reduced strength is a major factor in her ability to engage in the occupations she wants to do. Ms Tasker and the therapist need to determine if increasing her strength is possible or if she will have to adapt her occupations and environment to accommodate her reduced strength. This is a complex issue for Ms Tasker, because she lives a subsistence lifestyle in a community without any formal services. Changes in her life or adaptations to her environment, such as the purchase of a furnace and an oven to replace her woodstove, or connecting her home with electricity, would be beyond her personal financial means and would require outside resources.

Research in the area of human strength

Researchers have examined many different aspects of the importance of force, from the expected grip for individuals with rheumatoid arthritis[8] to adapted gait characteristics.[9,10] A number of groups of people, including children with cerebral palsy,[11] people who have experienced cerebral vascular accidents,[12] older individuals[13] and people with arthritis have been involved in studies to determine the amount and effect of the forces they can produce. Some of the results of those studies will be summarised briefly here. For further understanding of the work, it is recommended that therapists go to the primary sources, the journal articles, and read the research. The purpose of introducing the studies is to assure occupational therapists that there is research being conducted in kinetic analyses that will be useful to them in their practice. By studying and understanding the growing body of strength research in individuals with different physical difficulties, therapists will better be able to help people perform the occupations that they want to engage in.

Many children with cerebral palsy have been involved in research to enable therapists and others to understand and help to ameliorate their movement difficulties. For example, children with cerebral palsy have been given botulinum toxin A, and its effect on their muscle activity has been studied.[14] Toe walking patterns in children with cerebral palsy have also been studied.[15] Kinetic analysis has been used in the process of decision-making about surgery for these children.[11] Studies have been conducted to evaluate the effects of medical treatment and surgery.[16] Understanding these treatments for gait may help the future treatment of both upper and lower extremity function in children with movement difficulties and will improve the effectiveness of occupational therapy with these individuals.

It is difficult for an occupational therapist to determine with individuals who have had strokes if problems are due to muscle weakness or abnormal muscle tone. Individuals who have had strokes may have impaired reactions to external load disturbances in addition to weakness in their hands.[12]

For people who use wheelchairs, a number of issues have been examined using kinetic analyses. Awareness of force requirements of activities for wheelchair users can provide the occupational therapist with an indication of how much muscle strength or what torque requirements are needed for specific occupations. If therapists can use this information they might plan and implement exercise programmes and activities with the individual that will lead to the strength required. Researchers who have examined hand function and force in individuals who have had C_6 and C_7 spinal cord injuries have found that those individuals attain a good level of function, despite poor lateral force grasp in the hands.[17] Researchers have also examined the weight-relieving position of people who have C_5 and C_6 quadriplegia to determine the kinematics and kinetics involved in performing this action used to reduce pressure.[18]

Aging can negatively affect force production. Fingertip load force threshold in gripping has been found in older people and it appears to be consistent with degraded central information processing in older adults.[19] The implication for occupational therapists could be in providing appropriate adaptive devices for these individuals.

Force, as a measure of muscle function, is related to physical properties such as grip configurations,[20,21] forearm position,[21] and gait characteristics.[9,10,22] Force measurements are used as an input to systems, both mathematical and physical, to reproduce or understand force function. Information about force production has been used to design an artificial grasping system for a paralysed hand.[23,24] This information has also been used to introduce functional electrical stimulation into a treatment plan for individuals who have quadriplegia and weak hands.[25]

SYSTEMS OF FORCE

One force, be it from within the body or from machinery, does not work in isolation. There is resistance to exerted forces. For example, when a therapist teaches a person to use a reacher, the person must exert a force (sometimes called a motive or effort force) on the reacher, to open the reacher and hold it in position. This effort will be resisted by a spring or other component of some types of reachers which are designed to keep the reacher closed when the person loosens his or her grasp. This force can be exerted by a strong closing mechanism.

There will also be a resistance from the weight of any object being held above a surface, for example when lifting a hot pot in the kitchen. The resistance to movement is a force. A reacher closing mechanism, or the force of gravity holding a pot on the table, are both resistance forces that work against the force required for a movement. These forces that work against each other, or even forces working together to produce an action, are systems of forces. Ms Tasker must work against the weights or forces of objects all around her. She even has to strengthen the leg muscles that she has in the portion of her leg that was not removed, so that she can manipulate the prosthesis, which has a weight to it.

LEVER SYSTEMS

Lever systems of force have both effort and resistance forces. They usually have a point about which these forces act. This can be called an axis of rotation or a fulcrum. An example of a lever system is a teeter-totter or a board with a centre point about which the board rotates. Acrobats may use a specially designed board to perform the stunt where one person pushes down on one end while the other is sent into the air. The pushing acrobat is essentially the 'effort' or 'motive' force pushing onto the board. The other acrobat is the resistance. The acrobat producing the effort moves downwards, and exerts a force through the lever so that the acrobat at the other end is propelled upwards.

The designation of a lever system is based on the position of the effort force and the resistance in relation to the axis of rotation. The type of lever, quantity of these forces, and the distance they are from the axis of motion, all affect how the movement occurs. A lever system consists of at least two forces. A way to envision a simple lever system is to think of it as two forces: an effort or motive force and a resistive force. Both of these forces can be at the same distance from the axis of rotation. An example of a lever that we encounter in the occupational therapy domain is a manual feeding device that a person uses by pushing down with shoulder muscles. There is a pivot point somewhere along the length of the system. At the other end of the system is an eating utensil with food. The person guides the utensil to his or her mouth with the force exerted by muscle strength.

Levers can be very useful or they can make the effort required to move an object difficult. Whether or not a lever is useful can be determined by the type of lever it is, the distances the forces are from the axis, and the size or magnitude of the forces. A lever can increase a force, change the direction of the force application, or gain a distance from which to work, if distance is needed. The therapist who understands levers can use that knowledge in many ways. Understanding and using levers can help a therapist to determine the relative effectiveness of similar pieces of adaptive equipment and perhaps adapt the equipment so it is most effective for the person using it. Levers can also be used to advantage when designing splints.

Classes of levers

Levers are determined to be in one of three classes: first, second and third class. The class to which a lever belongs is determined by the location of the applied force (sometimes called the motive force), the resistive force and the fulcrum or axis of rotation.

There is another property of levers that affects how well they work, based solely on the distances that the forces are from the axis. This is called the mechanical advantage. Both the effort and the resistance are at a distance from the axis. The distance from the effort to the axis is called the force arm. The distance from the resistance to the axis is the resistance arm. Mechanical advantage is the force arm divided by the resistance arm. If, in the example of the acrobats on the teeter-totter, they both weigh the same amount and are the same distance from the central axis of the equipment, they will both sit in the air. If one of the acrobats moves back, thus increasing the distance from the axis, that acrobat will move down. The only difference is the increased distance from the axis. Using the equation for mechanical advantage, the effort arm is greater than the resistance arm, so the mechanical advantage is greater than 1.

First class levers

The axis of rotation is between the exerted force and the resistance force in a first class lever. Sometimes, the axis of rotation may be called the fulcrum, the exerted force may be called the effort force and the resistance force may be called the weight. Using equipment such as a crowbar is an example of a first class lever.

A pair of scissors is also a first class lever. The effort is exerted by the fingers, the axis is the point about which the scissors open and close, and the resistance is exerted by the person trying to open or close the scissors to cut an object. If the force exerted by the fingers is greater than the resistive force that might be represented by a piece of paper, then the paper will be cut. The paper will remain intact if the person does not have the strength to cut. The further the fingers are from the axis of rotation, the easier it will be to cut. So if a person has reduced strength due to a disability or injury, longer handles and a shorter distance between the axis and the cutting blades will make it easier to cut. In Figure 3.1 both pairs of scissors represent first class levers. Which pair of scissors would be easier to use and why? What other types of equipment are first class levers? Think of ways to make it easier for someone to use the equipment, based on the principles of a first class lever.

In a simple reaching device, if the axis of rotation is closer to the person holding the handles together, then the resistance arm is greater than the effort arm. This means the mechanical advantage is less than 1. If the axis is moved closer to the resistance, so that the effort arm length is greater than the resistance arm length, then the mechanical advantage is greater than 1. If the mechanical advantage is greater than 1, rather than less than 1, and

Figure 3.1 Scissors are first class levers.

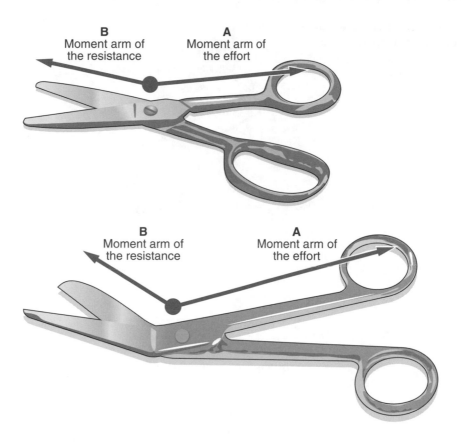

B
Moment arm of
the resistance

A
Moment arm of
the effort

B
Moment arm of
the resistance

A
Moment arm of
the effort

everything else stays the same, the activity should require less effort. A first class lever is the only class of lever that can have a mechanical advantage greater than or less than 1, depending on the position of the effort force as opposed to the resistance force.

Second class levers

In a second class lever system, the resistance force is always between the axis of rotation and the effort force. An example of a second class lever would be a wheelbarrow. The axis is the wheel, the resistance would be the weight, and the effort would be the person lifting the weight by the handles. In a second class lever system, the mechanical advantage is greater than 1, because the length of the effort arm is always greater than the length of the resistance arm, by definition. If someone is trying to lift something or move it, it will be easier to do using a second class lever than using a first class lever with a short effort arm relative to the resistance arm.

Using a piece of adapted cutting equipment in the kitchen is an example of a second class lever. In Figure 3.2, the axis is the point at which the knife tip is attached to the board. The resistance is exerted by whatever is cut, in this case an apple. The effort is exerted by the hand on the knife. The resistance arm is shorter than the effort arm, demonstrating a mechanical

Figure 3.2   Using a second class lever. A represents the effort arm, while B represents the resistance arm.

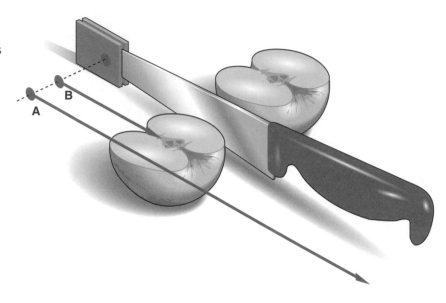

advantage greater than 1. A therapist who found that it was just a little too difficult for a person to cut using the knife could consider using a longer knife or moving the object to be cut closer to the axis. Either of these choices would increase the mechanical advantage. This is an example of why understanding the concept of mechanical advantage can be a tool for the therapist. Therapists can adapt equipment to make it more useful when they understand the concepts of mechanics.

Third class levers

A third class lever can be considered to work in the opposite way to a second class lever; the effort arm is always shorter than the resistance arm. The effort is between the axis of rotation and the resistance.

Lifting food to the mouth using a weighted spoon demonstrates use of a third class lever (see Fig. 3.3). The axis point is the ball at the end of the spoon. The effort is exerted at the hand, even though it may come from further up the arm. The resistance is the weight of the spoon and the weight of the food on it. No matter what the design, the effort will always be closer than the resistance to the axis of motion. How could you make it easier still for the child to lift the food?

More force must be exerted to overcome a load in a third class lever than in a second class lever. Most muscles in the body are third class levers, which means the muscle must exert more force than the resistance force is providing, in order for movement to occur. If you think that muscles being part of third class lever systems seem inefficient, you are right; it is. But there is a useful trade-off for this inefficiency. Muscles and the forces they work against being third class lever systems means that the muscle can be attached close to the axis of rotation. This closeness of attachment makes people a little more 'streamlined' than we would otherwise be.

Figure 3.3 Using a third class lever. **A,** from the weighted ball of the spoon to the hand, represents the effort arm; **B,** from the ball to the food on the spoon, represents the resistance arm.

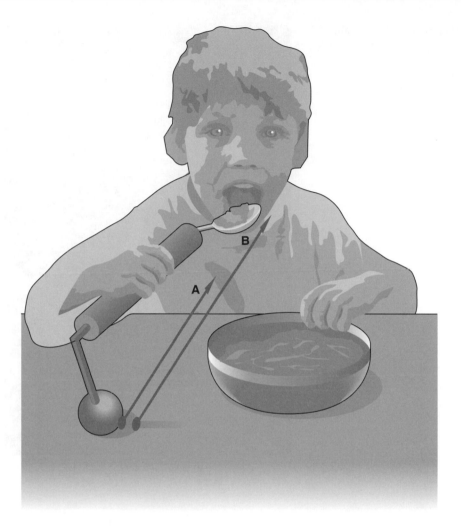

Example of a lever problem

When you are solving problems concerning levers to help someone perform a task more easily, you might want to draw a simple diagram and write down what you know about the problem, as described below.

You will want to know the values that you can measure. Then you can write down the equations. You then solve the equations and look at them. It is helpful to ask yourself if the numbers you have determined for the solution make sense with the rest of the numbers. For example, if most of the distances you are given are between 0.01 m and 0.05 m and your forces are also that small, but you come up with a number of 50 m, you may have made a mistake and will want to check your work.

Figure 3.4 gives you an opportunity to think through a lever problem using this method. What type of lever is this? Is the mechanical advantage greater than or less than 1? Lengths of the lever arms are given below.

Figure 3.4 The weight of the person's foot and leg (B) is being lifted by using the arms (C). The axis of the lever system is at A.

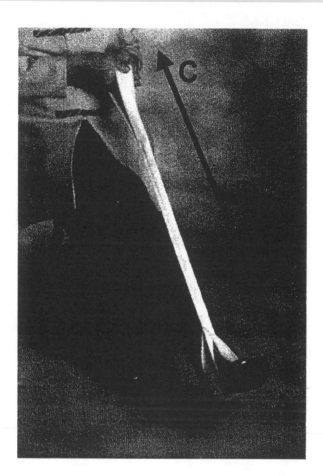

d_m = 500 cm (distance of the muscles, or the hand, to the axis of rotation)

wt = 100 N (weight of the leg)

d_{wt} = 200 cm (distance of the centre of the weight to the axis of rotation)

When you do a problem like this, it is always a good idea to draw a simple diagram. Also, write down the values that you know. Although we, as therapists, may not always know the exact location of muscle attachments, estimating the distances and forces may help us when we are doing therapy, for example, when we are adapting equipment.

The person holding the foot in Figure 3.4 is not moving at this time, so we say the problem is a static one. All the torques and forces at the joints must equal zero. Mathematically, this is described as

$$\Sigma T_e = 0$$

(This says that the sum of the torques at the elbow equals zero. We know this, because no movement is occurring and everything is in static equilibrium.) We know that the product (multiplication) of the force of the muscle and the distance between the muscle and the axis is positive, because it would move the leg in a counter clockwise direction (by convention). Counter clockwise is always considered positive in rotation. The product of the weight and its distance from the point of application is negative. If the weight were allowed to move the forearm, it would move it clockwise. Clockwise is always considered negative. So,

$$\Sigma T_e = (F_m)(d_m) - (wt)(d_{wt})$$

The one number we do not know, but would like to, is the force of the muscle. Since we know that $\Sigma T_e = 0$, we can then say that $0 = (F_m)(d_m) - (wt)(d_{wt})$. If we put the numbers that we know into the equation, we have:

$$0 = (F_m)(0.5 \text{ m}) - (100 \text{ N})(0.20 \text{ m}).$$

We change centimetres into metres because metres are the proper units to use, by generally accepted rules. Next, we find F_m by algebra:

$$(F_m)(0.5 \text{ m}) = (100 \text{ N})(0.20 \text{ m})$$

$$F_m = (\,(100 \text{ N})(0.20 \text{ m})\,)/0.5 \text{ m}$$

$$F_m = 40 \text{ Newtons.}$$

If we want to lighten a load for a person who has difficulty lifting during an occupation, we can use this example to give us an idea of what might make a difference. We know if we make the load lighter, or if we can shorten the distance between the load and the axis of rotation, we will probably make it easier for the person to perform the occupation.

COMPOSITION OF FORCES

Composition of forces means that we know two or more forces and we are trying to put them together into one force. This one force will then tell us what the total force is in a particular direction.

RESOLUTION OF FORCES

If we know the resultant force, we may want to find out how this force could be made up of two forces. We often try to find out what amount of the force goes along a bone. One portion of the force could cause bones to push against each other (called compression) or pull away from each other (called traction or tension) at a joint. The second part of the force might be at 90° or perpendicular to the bone and it will try to rotate the bone in the direction of the force.

In a forearm, the biceps muscle attaches at an angle to the lower arm. If we show the resolution of this force with forces perpendicular, or at right angles, to each other, we can have one part of the muscle force pulling into the joint causing joint compression. This compression can sometimes be useful to hold the joint together. The other part of the force will be at right angles to that force. If the biceps muscle contracts to bend the elbows without the opposing triceps muscle contracting, then the elbow joint will dislocate.

In the example of a finger sling for a hand splint shown in Figure 3.5, there is a force in the y direction (Fy). Fy means it is the force in the y direction, or by convention, upwards. There will also be a second part or component of the force that will be parallel along the finger. This component of the force will be in the x direction, or the side-to-side direction, and is called Fx. If the elastic is pulling on an angle, back towards the finger, the Fx component will be pulling back towards the finger and will work towards compressing the joint of the finger. If the elastic is pulling away from the

Figure 3.5 The diagrams show a finger in a sling which is part of a finger orthosis. The forces have been resolved into vertical (Fy) and horizontal (Fx) components.

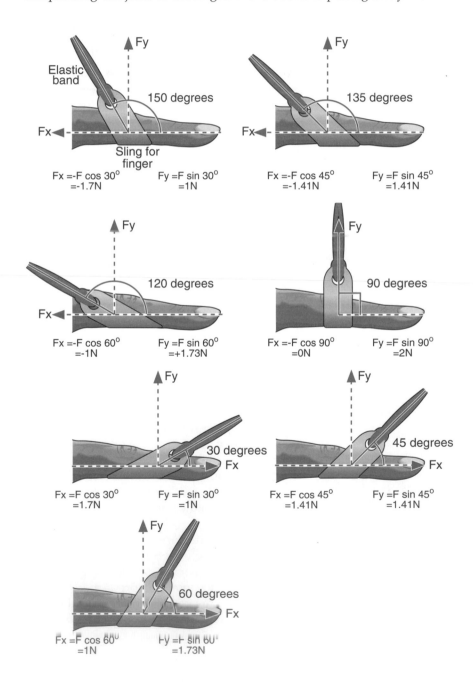

finger, there will still be a rotating component of the force. However, in this case, the parallel component (Fx) will be directed away from the finger and will be a distracting or traction force. The Fx force will be working to pull the bones apart at the joint. A therapist who wants to design a splint to pull upwards should put the splint elastic in a position that is as close to perpendicular to the finger as possible. This situation is described in Figure 3.5D. Look through Figure 3.5 and consider all the different forces occurring as a result of changing the angle of pull on the finger sling. It is not always possible to have the pull exactly the way you want for many reasons, such as swelling in the fingers, movement of the sling, and change in the position of the finger, but it is possible to try to approach the best possible position for the finger splint components. What is the effect of changing the sling's angle? What would be the best angle to use if you want all the force to be rotary or in the vertical direction?

Understanding forces and moments of forces or torques will help therapists design splints to do what they want them to do. Forces and torques are also used for many other applications, including the design of adaptive equipment and exercise programmes.

Another example of resolving forces can be evaluated when looking at slings for a person who has a flaccid hemiplegic shoulder. An analysis of this sling configuration demonstrates that part of the force at the affected elbow pulls up and a portion pulls towards the hand[26] (see Fig. 3.6). Different

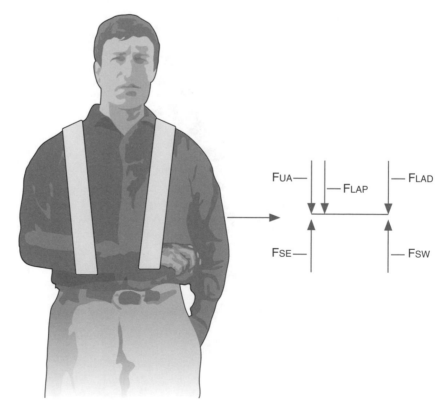

Figure 3.6   Figure 3.6(A) shows a splint over both arms. The forces, noted beside the diagram of the person, show that there is downward force on both the affected and unaffected shoulders.

Figure 3.6 *cont'd* The second sling (B) shows all the force over the unaffected shoulder.

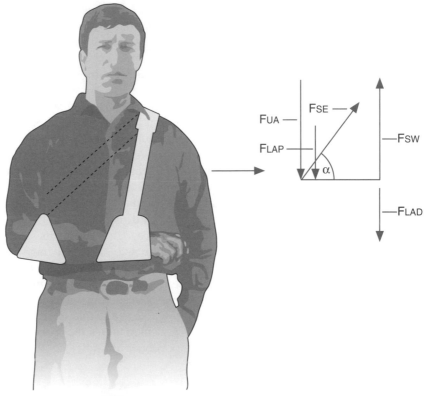

Figure 3.6 *cont'd* The third sling (C) shows a component of the force pushing the arm away from the body and force of the affected arm pulling directly downwards.

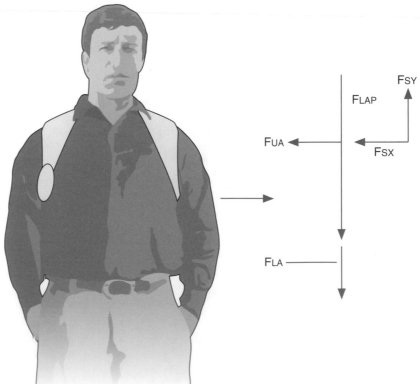

Figure 3.6 *cont'd* The fourth diagram (D) is a person resting his affected arm on a table. The table decreases the force on the arm, which is good, but is not practical for mobility purposes. (Adapted with permission of the Canadian Association of Occupational Therapists from Spaulding SJ, *Biomechanical analysis of four supports for the subluxed hemiparetic shoulder.* Can J Occup Ther 1999; 66(4):169–175.)[26]

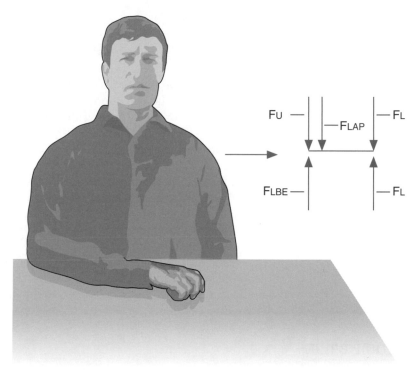

quantities of the forces shown are exerted up towards the shoulder, depending on the angle of the splint position. Which of these four support systems would you use? Would you decide to use no support? What would happen to the weight of the arm if you did not support it under any circumstances? There are no equations in this example, but there should be enough information for you to think about the problem of how or whether or not to ask a person who has experienced a stroke to use a sling or support system.

TORQUE

Torque is the product of a force and the perpendicular distance from the line of action of the force to the axis of rotation. This means the force may act at a distance from the object on which it is acting. This distance is called the perpendicular distance from the line of action of the force to the axis of rotation.

To get an idea of this concept, try tying a string to a door handle. Hang on to the end of the string and pull straight away from the door. The door should open easily. The string is acting as the moment arm, and shows the distance between the point of application (the door) and the force (your pull). If you move the string, so it lies closer to the hinges of the door, then pull, you will find it harder to open the door. It is more difficult to open the door because less of the force you are applying is pulling at right angles to the door.

In relation to Figure 3.5 a dynamic splint was used to explain the concept of the direction of pull of an elastic band. The same occupational therapy example can be used to understand torque as well. The elastic is attached to pull in the direction perpendicular to the attachment site on the splint. So the torque is pulling the finger into extension, if the elastics are on the dorsal side of the finger. The therapist must create the proper pull position and angle. Only then will the force and the torque on the finger be correct.

A counter clockwise torque, or pull, is defined to be positive. This is a convention. Whenever a person talks about a positive rotation, other people understand it to mean a rotation in a counter clockwise direction. A pull that causes a clockwise rotation is always negative. If a finger support elastic is pulling up as noted in Figure 3.5, and the observer looks at the sling, the pull of the elastic on the finger would be counter clockwise or in the positive direction. If we switched the picture around and the elastic seemed to pull in the clockwise direction, the force would be said to be pulling in the negative direction.

STATIC EQUILIBRIUM

If the system is motionless, it is said to be in a state of static equilibrium. The distance from the motive force to the axis, times the size of the motive force, will be equal to the distance of the resistive force times the size of the resistive force, so no movement can occur. This can happen, even if forces are working. For example, if someone is holding a spoon steady in their hand, with no movement, there must be some muscle action to hold the spoon up. There is also other muscle action working against that action, to hold the spoon steady. The steady spoon and the arm are said to be in static equilibrium.

DYNAMIC EQUILIBRIUM

A body or part of a body is in dynamic equilibrium if the forces on it are not equal. If the forces are not equal and do not add up to zero, then movement occurs. If there is movement, there is dynamic equilibrium.

SUMMARY

Kinetics is the term that describes forces and their relationships to movement. Therapists are often confronted with problems in which the individuals they work with cannot produce enough force to create movement or produce too much force, which is detrimental to the quality of movement. Individuals also deal with situations in which the equipment they use produces too little force to be functional or too much force so that occupations are hampered. By understanding kinetics a therapist has a new way of looking at the issues that the people they work with face, along with methods to enhance occupational performance.

QUESTIONS BASED ON THE CASE

1. What is the primary issue for Ms Tasker? Is there one overriding theme in her life that could be improved by her being able to increase her arm strength?
2. If Ms Tasker works hard at improving her arm force, but is unable to do any of the occupations she needs to do to live independently, how can the occupational therapist help her? Think of ways that the weights of objects in Ms Tasker's environment can be reduced, so she can use them more readily.
3. One issue that kept arising for Ms Tasker was mobility. Is there anything the therapist could recommend that would make Ms Tasker's ability to move around easier? Could any of her environments be adapted to meet her needs? Is there any type of mobility device that might be better for Ms Tasker than a manual wheelchair?
4. Ms Tasker's financial resources are limited. No matter how much the therapist wants to do to help Ms Tasker, or how much she herself wants to be involved in particular occupations, many suggestions will not be possible with her present income. Is there any source of income that you could tap, in the country in which you live, that could be used for Ms Tasker?·

Laboratory Exercise: Examples of Kinetics: the Implications of Adding Force during Occupations

1. Sit in a manual wheelchair, and have someone standing behind you to stop you if you begin to tilt in that direction. Try to push yourself up onto the back wheels. If you succeed, or even if you cannot do it, think about what type of lever you would represent. Think of the axis of the wheelchair and person combination as situated on the floor where the back wheels are in contact with the floor. If you lean too far back, the person behind you will have to catch you so you do not fall. If this happens, you have increased the amount of your weight and the weight of the wheelchair on one side of the axis.
2. Find a pair of crutches and use them with one of your legs off the ground. Move as quickly as you safely can, using the crutches. Be very aware of what is involved in stopping your movement. You have generated momentum as you have moved along. Is it difficult to stop? What kind of actions does it take to stop? Think about the force through your foot on the ground and through your hands to the crutches. Think about how much difficulty you might have if you had a lower extremity amputation as Ms Tasker has. How would that change what you can do? Sit with a partner and try to draw what the combination of a person and a pair of crutches would look like from the side. The axis of motion changes from the bottom of the foot to the crutches and back again. If you were working with Ms Tasker so she could do her occupations more confidently while she was using her crutches, are there things you could suggest to make her crutch use easier?

continued overpage

3. Find a piece of equipment, such as a reacher that is used to pick up objects or an adapted fork that has a curve in it, so it is easier to get it to a person's mouth. Consider the axis of the lever to be at the point at which you hold the object. If you add weight to the end of the equipment this will increase how much strength you need to lift the object. Is there a way, just by thinking of the lever arm of the equipment, to make the equipment easier to use? If you did not have enough strength, could you determine a programme that would increase your strength?

REFERENCES

1. Rodgers MM, Keyser RE, Gardner ER, Russell PJ, Gorman PH. Influence of trunk flexion on biomechanics of wheelchair propulsion. J Rehabil Res Dev 2000; 37:283–295.
2. White H, VandenBrink K, Augsburger S, Cupp T, Cottle W, Tylkowski C. Bilateral kinematic and kinetic data of two prosthetic designs: a case study. J Pediatr Orthop 2000; 12:120–126.
3. Hesse S, Luecke D, Jahnke MT, Mauritz KH. Gait function in spastic hemiparetic patients walking barefoot, with firm shoes, and with ankle-foot orthosis. Int J Rehabil Res 1996; 19:133–141.
4. Ounpuu S, Bell KJ, Davis RB III, DeLuca PA. An evaluation of the posterior leaf spring orthosis using joint kinematics and kinetics. J. Pediatr Orthop 1996; 16(3):378–384.
5. Cytowicz-Karpilowska W, Karpilowski B, Seyfried A. The influence of a joint orthosis on the grip force of the rheumatoid hand. Clin Rheumatol 1999; 18(5):373–384.
6. Stern EB. Grip strength and finger dexterity across five styles of commercial wrist orthoses. Am J Occup Ther 1996; 50(1):32–38. [erratum appears in Am J Occup Ther 1996 Mar; 50(3):193].
7. Alderson M, McGall D. The Alderson–McGall hand function questionnaire for patients with carpal tunnel syndrome: a pilot evaluation of a future outcome measure. J Hand Ther 1999; 12(4):313–322.
8. Fraser A, Vallow J, Preston A, Cooper RG. Predicting 'normal' grip strength for rheumatoid arthritis patients. Rheumatol 1999; 38(6):521–528.
9. Spaulding SJ, Patla AE, Elliott DB, Flanagan J, Rietdyk S, Brown S. Waterloo Vision and Mobility Study: gait adaptations to altered surfaces in individuals with age-related maculopathy. Optom Vis Sci 1994; 71(12):770–777.
10. Patla AE, Prentice SD, Robinson C, Neufeld J. Visual control of locomotion: strategies for changing direction and for going over obstacles. J Exp Psychol Hum Percept Perform 1991; 17(3):603–634.
11. DeLuca PA, Davis RB III, Ounpuu S, Rose S, Sirkin R. Alterations in surgical decision making in patients with cerebral palsy based on three-dimensional gait analysis. J Pediatr Orthop 1997; 17(5):608–614.
12. Grichting B, Hediger V, Kaluzny P, Wiesendanger M. Impaired proactive and reactive grip force control in chronic hemiparetic patients. Clin Neurophysiol 2000; 111(9):1661–1671.
13. Judge JO, Ounpuu S, Davis RB. Effects of age on the biomechanics and physiology of gait. Clin Geriatr Med 1996; 12:659–678.
14. Boyd RN, Pliatsios V, Starr R, Wolfe R, Graham HK. Biomechanical transformation of the gastroc-soleus muscle with botulinum toxin A in children with cerebral palsy. Dev Med Child Neurol 2000; 42:32–41.
15. Davids JR, Foti T, Dabelstein J, Bagley A. Voluntary (normal) versus obligatory (cerebral palsy) toe-walking in children: a kinematic, kinetic, and electromyographic analysis. J Pediatr Orthop 1999; 19(4):461–469.
16. Stefko RM, de Swart RJ, Dodgin DA, Wyatt MP, Kaufman KR, Sutherland DH, Chambers HG. Kinematic and kinetic analysis of distal derotational osteotomy of the leg in children with cerebral palsy. J Pediatr Orthop 1998; 18(1):81–87.

17. Harvey LA, Batty J, Jones R, Crosbie J. Hand function of C6 and C7 tetraplegics 1–16 years following injury. Spinal Cord 2001; 39(1):37–43.
18. Harvey LA, Crosbie J. Biomechanical analysis of a weight-relief maneuver in C5 and C6 quadriplegia. Arch Phys Med Rehabil 2000; 81(4):500–505.
19. Cole KJ, Rotella DL. Old age affects fingertip forces when restraining an unpredictably loaded object. Exp Brain Res 2001; 136(4):535–542.
20. Sharp WE, Newell KM. Coordination of grip configurations as a function of force output. J Mot Behav 2000; 32(1):73–82.
21. Richards LG, Olson B, Palmiter-Thomas P. How forearm position affects grip strength. Am J Occup Ther 1996; 50(2):133–138.
22. Rodgers MM, Mulcare JA, King DL, Mathews T, Gupta SC, Glaser RM. Gait characteristics of individuals with multiple sclerosis before and after a 6-month aerobic training program. J Rehabil Res Dev 1999; 36(3):183–188.
23. de Castro MCF, Cliquet A. An artificial grasping evaluation system for the paralysed hand. Medical and Biological Engineering and Computing 2000; 38(3):275–280.
24. Ferrari de Castro MC, Cliquet A. Artificial grasping system for the paralyzed hand. Artif Organs 2000; 24(3):185–188.
25. Davis SE, Mulcahey MJ, Betz RR. Making FREEHAND their hand: the role of occupational therapy in implementing FES in tetraplegia. Technol Disabil 1999; 11(1/2):29–34.
26. Spaulding SJ. Biomechanical analysis of four supports for the subluxed hemiparetic shoulder. Can J Occup Ther 1999; 66(4):169–175.

Chapter 4

Occupational therapy and mechanical principles

Mechanical principles have influence and come into play when we work with people who have physical problems. Mechanics can make our work easier and problem-solving more efficient. However, therapists are rarely, if ever, introduced to concepts such as stress, strain, damping or parallel elastic components of materials. In fact, I expect that many people who read this chapter will find these concepts new. The concepts they are familiar with, for example friction, will seem different, because they will be explained in more detail than therapists are used to.

These mechanical principles apply both to the workings of the body and to the equipment and materials we use while working with people. For example, a person can use springs to close an assistive device, such as a reacher. If two springs are put beside each other (in parallel), they will have a stronger elastic force than if one is attached to the end of the other one (in series).

When an occupational therapy student is learning how to use thermoplastic splinting material, the material often has to be reheated numerous times to produce the correct splint with good fit. For a student who is having difficulty or who is a bit of a perfectionist, the material may be reheated many times! Eventually, this material will stop being malleable, and will crack or break. The breaking of the material is an example of the property of the thermoplastic material. It eventually changes its mechanical properties and reaches what is called the ultimate failure point. The only option for the student practising with the material is to use a new piece of material.

The purpose of this chapter is to define and explain mechanical principles, such as spring characteristics and friction, and provide examples of some mechanical principles. Therapists will then know when to use them. A case study is provided to give the reader the opportunity to consider how to use some of the mechanical principles with a person they are working with.

CASE STUDY: MR DOUGLAS AZIZ

This is the case of Mr Douglas Aziz, a 73-year-old man who has retired from his position as a night watchman at a manufacturing company. He had held the position for approximately 35 years. Mr Aziz's retirement at 62 years of age was precipitated by some of the symptoms of Parkinson's disease. The disease was making it difficult for him to carry out his work. He was having difficulty walking as well as manipulating some of the equipment he needed to use during his work.

Mr Aziz goes to a clinic where the physician and therapy team specialise in neurological problems. The clinic is located about 200 km from his home, so he only attends once every 6 months; while he is there he usually has his medications adjusted, but does not participate in any occupational or physical therapy.

The settings

Mr Aziz lives with his wife in a small first-floor apartment of a house situated in a rural community. His landlord and landlady live upstairs. He would like to participate in some leisure activities but is finding the Parkinson's disease is limiting him.

The settings the occupational therapist will be working in with Mr Aziz are his home environment and the rural community. The apartment is small, but cheerfully decorated. Mr Aziz and his wife find that there is enough room for them. The community is in a hilly area, but most of the shops and buildings, such as the YMCA and the community centre, are close to the Aziz's home.

Mr and Mrs Aziz's grown children live very far away so there are no members of the family who are available to provide physical support for him. The family is definitely close emotionally, though. His children communicate regularly with their parents and visit about twice a year.

He and his wife have many friends, because they have been living in the community for much of his working his life and they both like to be sociable. They enjoy company and spending time with their friends. They like to play cards, go to movies, lawn bowl and swim at the local YMCA with their friends.

The occupational therapist

Ms Sonja Gibb has been an occupational therapist for about 20 years. She has held a number of different positions, including working within the school system, working in hand therapy, and now working with people who have neurological difficulties. She works in the community, through a community-based access centre and covers about a 300 km radius in her work. Now she works with older people who have had strokes, traumatic brain injury, multiple sclerosis and Parkinson's disease. She has started to work with Mr Aziz in the last 2 months, because of his concerns. She also knows that Mrs Aziz is doing many extra things to help her husband. Ms Gibb is concerned that Mrs Aziz is tiring more than she is willing to admit to her husband.

The individual

Mr Aziz is a very pleasant gentleman. He and his wife are quite happy together. Although he has retired, he stays in touch with some of the people from his work. He likes to go lawn bowling with his wife. He bowls with a group of friends who are quite comfortable with him taking longer to bowl than he once did. He also sits down to bowl, usually because his standing balance is not good enough for him to bowl standing up. Because he is with friends this is not a problem for the other people, many of whom are elderly. He also likes to play cards, although he is wondering if he will have to stop playing because he is finding it increasingly difficult to hold the cards. He is also finding that he has difficulty making himself understood while he is playing.

He loves to go with his wife on the train to visit his three daughters, all of whom live in a city about 250 km away. All of his daughters have children and he delights in interacting with his five grandchildren who are between the ages of 4 and 10. The daughters and their families also come to town when they can and stay with friends, because there is not enough room in the Aziz's apartment and it would also be too disruptive for them.

Physical abilities

Mr Aziz has had Parkinson's disease for approximately 15 years. In the last couple of years his medications have not been as effective as they used to be. He has pronounced dystonia in his hands. He has some difficulty walking and uses a walker most of the time. He freezes when he is walking and is often unable to walk through doorways. He has tremor and rigidity in his extremities. These movement problems are major. He knows that as time goes on these symptoms will cause him even more problems when he tries to engage in the occupations he wants to do. He feels he is becoming more limited by the physical problems associated with the disease.

Mrs Aziz has helped her husband with some of the activities he finds difficult, such as doing up buttons or tying his shoelaces. She goes with him when he is walking outside the home, because she is very aware of and concerned about his diminishing abilities. She is concerned when he tries to turn around to change direction when he is walking, because she sees how unsteady he is.

Emotional status

Mr Aziz is happily married. He is usually in good humour, but because of the disease he has difficulty showing facial expressions. He is having more difficulty with the disease lately, because he knows it is affecting him more, and he finds he gets depressed at times. He certainly has accommodated his occupations to the physical difficulties and has made a conscious effort to enjoy his life, his family and his friends. In the last year or two he has been finding that he has been unable to deal with the disease as easily as he used to handle it. He and his wife have accepted the disease and they are trying to get on with their lives as best they can. Up until recently, they have been managing well. Mrs Aziz is having difficulty right now, because it is hard for her to see her husband unhappy and having so many problems.

EXPLORING ISSUES WITH MR AZIZ

Issues for Mr Aziz are directly related to his increasing physical difficulties. There are also problems with communication because he is having difficulty articulating and cannot always be understood. He finds that the tremor in his upper extremities makes eating and taking care of himself difficult and time-consuming. His wife is doing more for him.

He is finding that his ability to participate in activities around the house, as he always has done, is severely limited. However, this does not stop him from wanting to contribute or being involved in household activities. These contributions seem to him to be good things to do, but his wife is becoming increasingly concerned about him.

The occupational therapist who met briefly with the Azizs when they were last at the clinic thought that they might benefit from some help from a local occupational therapist in the community. They agreed. The main reason Mr Aziz contacted the occupational therapist, on this recommendation, was to take a good look at his occupations to see where he could benefit from help. He also wants to deal with his unhappiness about his difficulties. He does not want to give up his leisure activities, but is really worried that he might have to stop doing things.

FUNDAMENTAL CONCEPTS OF SOME MECHANICAL PRINCIPLES

Many mechanical principles will be defined and described in this chapter. Some of the principles will be useful for Mr Aziz and others will not. All of the principles, however, are ones that can be used by occupational therapists to make occupations easier, to understand how equipment works, or to design and change adaptive equipment for individuals.

- *Friction:* Friction is a force that is present at the contact point between two surfaces. Friction is composed of the downward force or weight of one object on another and the coefficient of friction.[1] The coefficient of friction is a number that represents the characteristics of the surfaces that are in contact with one another. Friction, then, is the weight of an object divided by the coefficient of friction.

  The equation for friction is:

  $$F_m = \mu_s N$$

  where F_m is the maximum value of the force, μ_s is the coefficient of static friction and N is the normal force or force acting straight downward on an object.
  - *Static friction:* Static friction is equal to the normal force of the object (that is, the direct downward force) times the coefficient of friction.
  - *Dynamic friction:* Dynamic friction is the friction that is produced when there is movement between two surfaces. Usually, in occupational therapy, there will be movement of a person or object on a surface. The equation for dynamic friction is:

    $$F_k = \mu_d N$$

  where F_k is the kinetic or dynamic friction, μ_d the coefficient of dynamic friction and N is the normal or downward force action on the object. If a pull is exerted on an object on a surface, it will eventually become strong enough that it will make the object move then it becomes easier to move the object. The force to keep something moving is always less than the force required to start it moving.
- *Pressure:* Pressure is force divided by surface area.

  $$P = F/A$$

  where P is the pressure, F is the force and A is the area over which the force is exerted.
- *Springs:* Springs store energy when they are stretched. When they are released from the stretched position, they move back into a position of rest. A spring's stored energy is directly related to its change in length or it can be considered to be related to its change in displacement. In other words the force exerted by a spring is related to the length of the spring when it is stretched times the spring constant, which is expressed in Newtons per metre
  The equation for a spring force is:

$$F = kx$$

where F is the force exerted by the spring, k is the spring constant and x is the change in the length of the spring from its resting position.

■ *Viscous damping:* In mechanics, a damper is considered to store energy. 'Viscous damping is characterized by the fact that the friction force is directly proportional to the speed of the moving body.'[2] In other words, if you pull two parts of a damper (for example, a type of bicycle pump) it requires more force to move it if it is moved quickly than if it is pulled apart slowly.

■ *Stress:* Stress is the 'load, or force, per unit area that develops on a plane surface within a structure in response to externally applied loads.'[3] The units of stress are N/m².

■ *Strain:* 'Strain is the deformation (change in dimension) that develops within a structure in response to externally applied loads.'[3] Strain can either be linear, in which a material is lengthened or shortened or it can be shear, which is the amount of angular change.

■ *Elasticity*: Elasticity is a property of materials. If a material is elastic, it returns to its original length and shape after it is stretched. Figure 4.1 shows elasticity in a spring weight. As the woman puts the tea leaves she has picked into the basket, the spring loaded scale above it is pulled down by the force of gravity. The more leaves the basket holds, the greater will be the number shown on the scale. Can you remember the value for the acceleration due to gravity?

If two elastics or springs are put side by side (in parallel), their strength is added together. This is illustrated in Figure 4.2. The elastic or rubber bands can be considered to be springs in parallel. How could you increase the force required to pull the handle? How much would the total force of the elastics change if you added two elastics? How much would it change if you took one elastic off? If they are attached with one end of one spring attached to the end of the other one (in series), then the force of the springs is divided by two.

■ *Plasticity:* A plastic material is one in which there is no elasticity or no give. A completely plastic material will break if force is exerted on it.

■ *Vibration or tremor:* Vibration is a very fast repetitive motion that can be found in equipment. 'A mechanical vibration is the motion of a particle or a body which oscillates about a position of equilibrium.'[2] Sometimes you can feel a vibration from the engine of a car if you put your hand on the outside of the car when it is running. An elastic band vibrates if one person holds each end and someone else pulls it in the middle, then the person holding it in the middle lets it go.

Tremor is also an oscillatory or repetitive motion. We think of earthquakes as tremors. Some people with neurological problems will also have a tremor in their muscles. The tremor shows up if you watch them move (this is called an intention tremor) or when they are quiet (called a resting tremor). A tremor is sometimes modelled or explained as a wave. A wave goes up and down. People can shake, or show a tremor, at between 8 and 12 times a second. The unit of a tremor or wave is called a Hertz (Hz). One Hz is one cycle per second. So a person can have an intention tremor of 12 Hz. Clonus, which is also a tremor, is slower and can sometimes be seen in people who have had spinal cord injuries. Clonus occurs at about 6 Hz.

Figure 4.1 Spring weight using gravity.

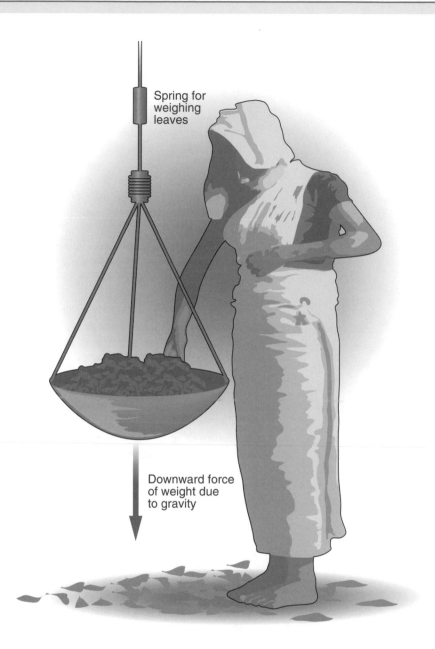

Spring for weighing leaves

Downward force of weight due to gravity

FRICTION

The weight of an object is always considered to be directed downwards because the object is being pulled down by gravity. If the object is on a sloped surface, for example a person sitting on a chair with a sloped seat, the only part of the person's weight that will go into the friction equation will be the weight going directly downwards. This makes sense. Think about the person sitting on the chair. If the chair tilts, the person may slide off, so the component of their weight directed through the chair seat has decreased so much that sliding out of the chair occurs.

Figure 4.2 Finger exerciser used to strengthen the fingers.

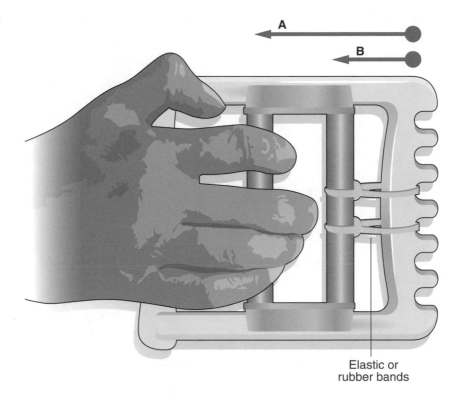

Elastic or
rubber bands

The coefficient of friction is based on the surface characteristics of the two surfaces that are in contact. If the surfaces are both rough, like sandpaper, rough-soled shoes, or a rough ground surface, then the coefficient of friction will be high. Researchers have worked to determine the coefficient of friction under different circumstances.[4] The highest number for the coefficient of friction is 1. If the two surfaces are very smooth, like ice and very shiny-bottomed shoes, then the coefficient of friction will be small and may approach zero. In this case, there is a chance of the person slipping on the ice when walking. People intuitively make adjustments to lower friction under their feet. For example, they may change the first step when they start walking, to decrease the chances of slipping.[5] Older adults adapt their gait during stair descent to accommodate to frictional characteristics.[6]

Friction can help or hinder. In Figure 4.3 the child stays upright because the force exerted downwards and the friction coefficient between the skate blade and the ice are adequate. What would happen if the coefficient of friction was lower? Adjustments to friction can be used when a person has reduced strength and needs to slide an object. For example, if a person were trying to move a cooking pot along a kitchen counter, it would be very difficult if the pot and the counter were both rough. It would be made easier if the pot had a smooth bottom and the counter were slippery. The movement would be easier still if the pot were put on a tray that had rollers on the bottom of it to roll it along the counter.

Figure 4.3 Friction helps the child remain standing on skates.

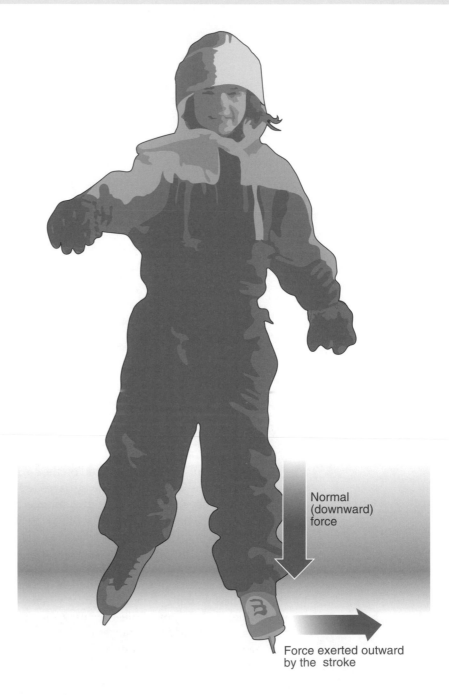

Normal (downward) force

Force exerted outward by the stroke

Friction can be a problem in walking.[7–10] Friction is important when considering the foot's contact with the ground. The coefficient of friction has also been studied during walking in individuals who have experienced cerebral vascular accidents and during walking on slippery versus non-slippery surfaces.[8–11] Researchers[5] found for young, healthy subjects, that if the friction was low between the foot and the floor during the initiation of walking, they would decrease the step length of the first step to deal with the low friction on the ground. Friction is a problem during transfers, particularly during sliding transfers from one surface to another. Sliding in rough clothing along a surface can cause skin breakdown. Friction-reducing devices can reduce the burden on care givers who are doing transfers.[12]

Interfaces between a person's skin and prosthesis, orthoses, equipment or tools impact function. A good interface can be crucial for skin integrity and reducing pain.[13,14] The interface between the lower-limb prosthesis and the limb has been used to evaluate comfort and function.[15] A functional handgrip test has been used to determine the static coefficient of friction between the hand and a handle.[4] Friction reduction has also been addressed by people providing products to athletes, in order to help reduce skin friction and resultant breakdown.[13] Friction has been measured indirectly in determining the friction surrounding tendons in fingers.[16]

PRESSURE

Pressure is the force exerted over an area. If you have the same force but applied over a large area, there will be a decrease in pressure. Horses exert a huge amount of pressure on the ground when they walk, because they put a large amount of weight through a small area. Too much pressure on the skin can result in skin problems, some of which can be serious. If there is too much pressure, because the person is bony and puts much of their weight through a bony prominence, or because a seating system is not properly prescribed, skin breakdown can occur. Pressure ulcers can be a serious concern for people who have insensate or delicate skin. They may not know how to relieve pressure or they may have come in contact with something that is causing pressure and not know it. Interface pressure has been evaluated for its role in soft tissue breakdown.[17]

Pressure can be reduced by increasing the surface area over which a force is exerted.[18,19] For example, good wheelchair cushions allow the force exerted on the seat by a person to be spread out over a large area. Another example is gloves that have been designed to decrease the effects of pressure.[20]

VIBRATION

Vibration is the very fast repeated movements that can be felt under many circumstances. A jackhammer (that is, a piece of machinery used by hand that can be used to cut concrete) produces vibration that can be felt up the arms. Exposure to periods of vibration, either to part of the body, or to the whole body, can negatively involve function. Vibration has been found to affect a person's performance negatively. Designs and modelling used to understand the effects of vibration have been used to provide information for the design of equipment, such as seating systems.[21]

Tremors, particularly intention tremors, make movement difficult. Can you imagine trying to eat when your hand is always shaking? Medications can help some tremors. If you think of a wave, it has a height (amplitude) and occurs over again at a certain rate (frequency). One thing we do know, that may help people reduce the effect of tremor, is that by adding weight to the arm we can reduce the amplitude of the tremor, but this will not have an effect on the frequency of the tremor. Wrist weights may help to dampen a tremor. Clonus can be brought to a stop by slowly stretching out a muscle, because clonus is not modulated by the brain, but by the muscle spindle and reflexes associated with it.

DAMPING

A damper (or dashpot as it is sometimes called) is dependent on the velocity of movement. It is often a property of liquids. For example, blood in the muscle can be thought of as having damping properties. Damping has been evaluated in relation to wheelchair use.[22]

VISCOELASTICITY

An object that has viscoelastic properties has the properties of both a viscous damper and a spring. Such an object will respond both to a change in its length and to the speed at which change occurs. A muscle is viscoelastic. It responds to both stretch and the speed of stretch.

STRESS AND STRAIN

An object, such as a tissue in the human body,[23] may be loaded or stressed. When it is stressed, there will probably be a change in it. Strain or deformation occurs. If the object is elastic and the load is taken off, then the object will return to its original length. If there is also a plastic region and the object is not stressed strongly enough to break it, then it will not break but it will not return to its original shape. If it is stressed even more strongly, the material will reach a failure point and break.

Therapists who work with splinting material work with thermoplastic materials. When the materials are heated, they can be changed in shape, and that shape is held once the materials cool down. Splinting material is plastic – it does not return to its original shape after it is loaded. If it is worked enough, it may break. Some splinting materials are said to have a memory. These materials will return to their original shape. They have elasticity in them. Splinting materials are not simple, because these changes are based on temperature.

Bones have the property of plasticity. If enough load or stress is placed on the bone with enough strength, it will not bend but will break. Tendons have elasticity in them and will spring back into position under a load, but if more stress is placed on them, they may deform and not return to their original length. Therapists who stretch out joints that have contractures and hold them stretched, either by holding them or splinting them, are working on the principle of plasticity in the tissues. Holding them out for a long enough time will cause them to stay lengthened. The therapists' problem, which cannot be solved here, is how much force to apply. How long to apply the force for optimal stretch or contracture depends on the needs of the individual. We know that stress over time will cause a change in structures.

SUMMARY

There are many mechanical principles that are present when we do occupational therapy. We often use these principles successfully without fully realising that the principles have specific definitions. Understanding more about the principles helps us to use them more effectively and to use them to our advantage when we are working with people who have physical problems.

QUESTIONS BASED ON THE CASE

1. Parkinson's disease can be, and usually is, progressive. Mr Aziz appears to be functioning quite well with it right now. Find out what you can about the disease process and its underlying causes, and speculate on what difficulties might present themselves to Mr Aziz in the future. Given those difficulties, what type of adaptive equipment for his self-care, instrumental activities of daily living, and leisure activities would you recommend?
2. Many mechanical principles have been described in this chapter, including friction, stress, strain and vibration. How would these principles apply to the adaptive equipment that you could recommend for Mr Aziz?
3. What occupations will Mr Aziz be able to do and which ones might he have to stop doing now? Are there any safety issues related to these occupations that could be addressed to make it easier for him to do them?
4. It has been noted that Mr Aziz is on a limited income. He has not described this as a problem; however, it may limit the amount of equipment he can buy. He does have a couple of very good friends who are both woodworkers and work in metal. Are there any pieces of adaptive equipment that you could design and have made by his friends, so that the equipment could then be used by Mr Aziz? Be sure that where you work is an area in which it is acceptable for occupational therapists to be involved in equipment design.
5. Mr Aziz's wife is quite physically fit and is very willing to help Mr Aziz when he needs it. Would you suggest that she become involved with his physical needs at this time? Is there a need for it in the future?

Laboratory Exercise: Examples of Mechanical Principles Applied to Improve Occupational Performance

1. A number of mechanical principles have been described in this chapter. You as a therapist or an occupational therapy student may have access to adaptive equipment or adaptive equipment catalogues. Look at the equipment or the book. Can you determine some of the mechanical characteristics of these pieces of adaptive equipment that make them useful for the individual? For example, if you are working in a paediatrics clinic and find a piece of

continued overpage

dycem, or non-slip material of some sort, can you find a use for it because of its property of increasing friction with the object with which it is in contact? Can you think of a situation in which a piece of adaptive equipment increases friction and therefore becomes a problem?

2. You may be considering helping someone strengthen their upper extremities using theraband. If you have only one level of elasticity of theraband available to you, how can you increase the strength with which the theraband can act on the person? Would you consider putting the theraband in parallel strips? Would you lengthen the theraband? Would you request that the individual stretch the theraband out farther, or not as far?

3. An issue which occurs in occupational therapy clinics, or in practice, is the desire to incorporate mechanical principles into occupations. Can you think of occupations within your clinical setting, or a setting you have visited, that can be adapted using mechanical principles? For example, one of the most complex areas in which to work in a home is in the kitchen. There are a great many different physical requirements to perform cooking and cleaning tasks.

   a. How might you consider adapting these? Consider the concept of friction and reducing or increasing friction as it is needed. Consider, also, all the other mechanical principles described in this chapter.

   b. To make it more specific for yourself, choose one activity. If you, yourself perform this activity, do the activity and describe it. Think of somebody who requires strengthening activities. Can you adapt the same task so that someone would be required to increase force output to do the task? Think of some other occupation in which you are involved. Can you change the occupation so that it is easier or more difficult for someone to do?

REFERENCES

1. Chang W-R. The effects of slip criterion and time on friction measurements. Safety Science 2002; 40(7–8):593–611.
2. Beer FP, Johnston ER. Vector mechanics for engineers. 4th edn. New York: McGraw-Hill; 1984.
3. Nordin M, Frankel VH. Basic biomechanics of the musculoskeletal system. 2nd edn. Philadelphia: Lea & Febiger; 2004.
4. O'Meara DM, Smith RM. Functional handgrip test to determine the coefficient of static friction at the hand/handle interface. Ergonomics 2002; 45(10):717–731.
5. Asaka T, Saito H, Yoshida N, Urakami D, Kamada K, Fukushima J. Relationship between the required coefficient of friction and gait initiation in young adults on a low friction floor. J Phys Ther Sci 2002; 14(1):33–39.
6. Christina KA, Cavanagh PR. Ground reaction forces and frictional demands during stair descent: effects of age and illumination. Gait Posture 2002; 15(2):153–158.
7. Burnfield JM, Tsai J, Souza R, Popovich J, Powers CM. Comparison of coefficient of friction requirements during level walking and stair descent in persons with and without a cerebral vascular accident. J Geriatr Phys Ther 2002; 25(3):25.
8. Cham R, Redfern MS. Heel contact dynamics during slip events on level and inclined surfaces. Safety Science 2002; 40(7–8):559–576.
9. Cham R, Redfern MS. Changes in gait when anticipating slippery floors. Gait Posture 2002; 15(2):159–171.
10. Myung R. Use of backward slip to predict falls in friction test protocols. Int J Ind Ergon 1 Nov 2003; 32(5):341–348.

11. Powers CM, Burnfield JM, Lim P, Brault JM, Flynn JE. Utilized coefficient of friction during walking: static estimates exceed measured values. J Forensic Sci 2002; 47(6):1303–1308.
12. Bohannon RW. Losing friction: the burden on caregivers during transfers can be greatly eased by friction-reducing devices. Rehab Manage 2003; 16(3):26–28.
13. Brueck CM. The role of topical lubrication in the prevention of skin friction in physically challenged athletes. J Sports Chiropract Rehabil 2000; 14(2):37–43.
14. Sivamani RK, Goodman J, Gitis NV, Maibach HI. Friction coefficient of skin in real-time. Skin Res Technol 2003; 9(3):227–233.
15. Mak AFT, Zhang M, Boone DA. State-of-the-art research in lower-limb prosthetic biomechanics–socket interface: a review. J Rehabil Res Dev 2001; 38(2):161–173.
16. Schweizer A, Frank O, Ochsner PE, Jacob HAC. Friction between human finger flexor tendons and pulleys at high loads. J Biomech 2003; 36(1):63–71.
17. Lowthian P. Measurement of interface pressure and its role in soft tissue breakdown. J Tissue Viability 2003; 13(2):80.
18. Sprigle S. Effects of forces and the selection of support surfaces. Top Geriatr Rehabil 2000; 16(2):47–62.
19. Stinson MD, Porter-Armstrong A, Eakin P. Seat-interface pressure: a pilot study of the relationship to gender, body mass index, and seating position. Arch Phys Med Rehabil 2003; 84(3):405–409.
20. Muralidhar A, Bishu RR. Safety performance of gloves using the pressure tolerance of the hand. Ergonomics 2000; 43(5):561–572.
21. Rosen J, Arcan M. Modeling the human body/seat system in a vibration environment. J Biomech Eng 2003; 125(2):223–231.
22. Kauzlarich JJ, Bruning TE III, Thacker JG. Wheelchair caster shimmy II: damping. J Rehabil Res Dev 2000; 37(3):305–313.
23. Chaffin DB, Stump BS, Nussbaum MA, Baker G. Low-back stresses when learning to use a materials handling device. Ergonomics 1999; 42(1):733–736.

Chapter 5

Motor control and motor learning: acquiring skills for occupational performance

Motor control and motor learning are not classified under biomechanics by most people in the discipline. However, occupational therapists who work with individuals who have movement difficulties are always watching motion and how people learn movements. They are also often involved in teaching movements. There is an extensive body of literature that describes how people control and learn movements. Most of the work on this that was done in the past related to people who did not have physical difficulties, but now more research is being done that evaluates movement in the people with difficulties with whom therapists work.

The ability to control motor activities and the ability to learn new activities are both essential to physical and social wellbeing as well as to participation in occupations. Without the ability to control movement and learn new skills, people would be unable to engage effectively in occupations, including activities of daily living, work and leisure. Learning movement skills is dependent on the control characteristics of the individual, the environment in which the person learns, and the attributes of the skills which make up occupations. Superimposed on these individual domains is the interaction between the learner, the environment and the occupation.

This interaction between learner, environment and occupation also includes the person who enhances the learning process when intervention or training occurs. In the case of rehabilitation, the therapy student or therapist would engage in helping a person learn a task. Individual learning is an integral part of rehabilitation. The individual and the therapist work as a team, to enable the individual to learn the skills that compose the occupations that the individual wants to engage in.

This chapter will describe current knowledge about motor learning and motor control, and will introduce the literature, addressing specific learning paradigms and their effects on people who need to learn new skills or relearn skills because of changes in their motor control status.

The chapter will focus on observed characteristics of learned skills. The goals of the chapter are to explain the components of human movement and to help the therapist consider these aspects in order to assist individuals to learn tasks which come together to become physical occupations. Biomechanical analyses of movement will be described only where they are essential to understanding the context for movement.

CASE STUDY: MS JOAN SPIEGEL

Ms Joan Spiegel is a 50 year old woman who has been living alone for the last 10 years. She has never been married and does not have children. She has been a successful solicitor who has worked her way up through the corporate structure of a large law firm and was a senior partner in the firm when she sustained a left cerebral vascular accident (CVA).

The setting

Ms Spiegel was stabilised in an acute care facility and has now been transferred to a long-term rehabilitation facility, located in the downtown area of the city where she lives. Her apartment is about half an hour away from the hospital by car and longer by public transport.

The occupational therapy department is equipped with assessment tools and up-to-date rehabilitation equipment. The rehabilitation staff include an attending physician, physiotherapist, social worker, psychologist, speech therapist and occupational therapist.

The occupational therapist

The occupational therapist, Ms Gail Atkins, has 15 years experience working with adults in various rehabilitation settings. She has worked with a number of people who have experienced CVAs. She has been working with Ms Spiegel for a week but has seen little progress in Ms Spiegel's motor abilities and expects that the rehabilitation will take a relatively long time and that changes will come about slowly.

The individual

Ms Spiegel has always been driven to do well in her chosen work. She has left herself little time for leisure activities, family or friends. The only leisure time she spends is reading a novel once in a while and travelling every couple of years for about 2 weeks. She has been a successful lawyer and had planned to continue with this work.

Physical abilities

Ms Spiegel sustained a severe left CVA of the middle cerebral artery 4 weeks ago. She has just been transferred from the acute care unit of the general hospital to the rehabilitation hospital and is medically stable enough to begin the initial phases of rehabilitation.

After a week with Ms Spiegel, the occupational therapist has found that she has many difficulties. She has problems in all the physical, cognitive and affective areas. More specifically, she has the following difficulties: a dense (very flaccid) right hemiplegia, low tone throughout the right side, pain in her right shoulder, dysarthria, and very little sensation. Ms Spiegel lacks deep and light touch, as well as kinaesthesia and proprioception.

She is almost totally dependent on others to take care of her physical needs right now. She is not close to considering if she will be able to return to work.

Emotional status

Ms Spiegel is very depressed. Based on information from her family, the psychiatrist and the psychologist, her depression does not seem to predate her CVA but is considered to be a reaction to having had the CVA. The health professionals on the rehabilitation team are monitoring the depression, talking with Ms Spiegel, and considering discussing with her the possibility of taking medication for the depression in the short term. It is not surprising to anyone that she might be depressed, because the CVA was a heavy blow to her and has removed her ability to take care of herself, on top of stopping her career in its tracks.

Exploring issues with Ms Spiegel

The issues for Ms Spiegel are extremely complex. She is most concerned about her career, as it was the main occupation by which she identified herself. On a daily basis she is also frustrated by her lack of ability to take care of herself, which she finds humiliating. She does not like her life being out of her control and feels devastated by the CVA.

At the end of the chapter, there are questions pertaining to this case. You might want to refer back to the case as you are reading the material, so that you can answer the questions.

FUNDAMENTAL CONCEPTS FOR UNDERSTANDING MOTOR CONTROL AND MOTOR LEARNING

- *Motor control:* Motor control is the observed and measurable motor activity.
- *Motor learning:* Motor learning is the change in motor function that is retained over time.
- *Feedback:* This is information provided to oneself when learning and working on a task.
- *Fitt's law:* There is an inverse relationship between speed and accuracy. Accuracy decreases as speed increases. Also, if speed decreases, accuracy increases.
- *Knowledge of results:* Knowledge of results is the provision of information to a person about performance. This information is not available from the person's own sensory systems.

MOTOR CONTROL AND LEARNING

Motor control is an area of study that evaluates perceived movement and attempts to understand the mechanisms, including physiological, cognitive and biomechanical, that underlie the movement. Motor learning represents the changes that allow motor skills to occur and be retained over time. The process of acquiring motor learning, which cannot be seen or measured, can be contrasted with motor behaviour, which is observable and measurable motor activity. Figure 5.1 illustrates an activity acquired by successful motor learning. The child has played with a hula hoop often enough to be able to walk, look around and keep the hoop up at the same time. How would you teach someone to do this? What steps of training would you use?

Therapists benefit from an understanding of motor control and motor learning, because this knowledge provides them with tools to teach motor skills. Understanding of these processes is increasing as applied researchers further explore the ability of individuals to learn new tasks and learn about what sources to tap to enhance learning for the individuals with whom they work.

Figure 5.1 Child with a hula hoop.

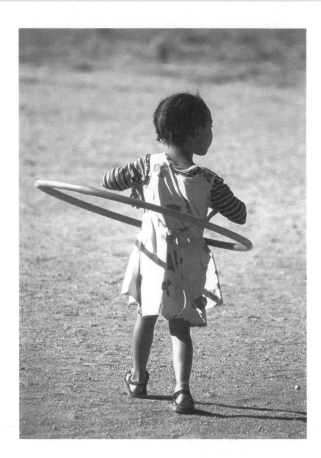

BEHAVIOUR CLASSIFICATION

Successful motor function can be dependent on characteristics of the behaviour being evaluated. Motor behaviour can be classified as: open or closed; discrete, serial, or continuous; and simple or complex.

Open and closed skills

An open skill is one that can respond to a changing environment, although there can be a plan to execute a movement even within a changing environment. An example would be propelling a wheelchair on an accessible walkway in the woods. The path can be smoothed to ensure that the wheels will not stick, but the path may meander, curve and include inclines and declines. Weather, including temperature changes, the amount of available light, and precipitation, will all potentially influence the progression of the wheelchair user. Driving a car using hand controls is another example of an open task. The driver, like the person propelling the wheelchair, is required to take note of and respond to the environment.

Closed skills are characterized by predictable environments. Brushing one's teeth and combing one's hair in a familiar bathroom at home are closed skills. The implements required to complete the tasks are in known places and there are no unpredictable environmental changes to which the person needs to adapt. Open skills are skills that can occur in random environments. An example of a random environment would be a busy street in a large city. It is difficult to know the speed of the traffic or the planned activities of individual drivers.

Discrete and continuous skills

On the continuum of discrete to continuous skills, discrete skills are ones that are completed once and have a noticeable beginning and ending. An example of a discrete skill would be doing a transfer from a bed to a bathtub. Other examples are repeated skills, such as buttoning a shirt with a button hook or using a sock aid, that require discrete actions to be strung together. Figure 5.2 gives another example of a discrete skill. The boy's basketball practice is made easier by the position and size of the basket. Note the requirements of the movement: he must balance on his toes; extend his arms to release the ball on the right angle; and watch the hoop as he is doing the activity. Formulate some ideas that will make tasks challenging, but possible, for individuals with whom you work.

A continuous skill is one where the individual continues doing a task until choosing a stopping point in time. There is no set recognisable beginning or end to a continuous skill. Steering an electric scooter along a path or in a shopping mall requires continuous control of movement and can include making adjustments throughout the activity.

Simple and complex skills

Simple skills consist of very few components. A simple skill for someone who does not have upper extremity motor difficulties is brushing one's teeth. A complex skill is one in which there are many components to be learned and remembered; for example, some of the t'ai chi moves are very complex and take a long time to learn well.

HOW TO MEASURE AND UNDERSTAND MOTOR BEHAVIOUR

Skills can be measured by evaluating the biomechanical characteristics of the movements required by the skills, the accuracy of the movement, and the speed of the movement. Accuracy is measured in simple tasks by determining how close one comes to reaching to a specified target or how closely a movement follows a predetermined path. Speed can be measured by determining reaction time, or how quickly a person initiates a response to a stimulus to move. Movement time is the time between the initiation of a response and the end of the response. Pooling together reaction time and movement time provides a measure of the total time.

Fitt's law describes the relationship between speed and accuracy. The trade-off between speed and accuracy dictates that if the speed of a movement increases, then accuracy decreases. For example, a person in a sitting position is asked to reach a point on a communication board quickly.

Figure 5.2 Practising a basketball throw.

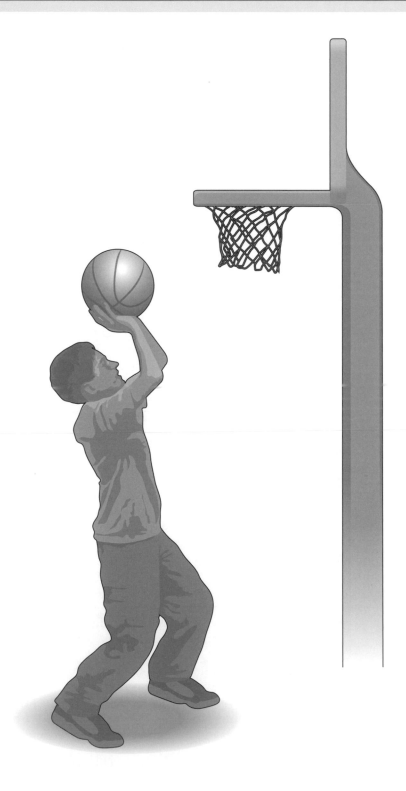

This demands that the person does the movement with speed. Someone who is still learning to use the board may not be able to move to the required position quickly, but may be able to reach the intended position if asked to slow down. In this example, the person can either move quickly and not touch the required spot or move slowly and reach it. The person cannot move quickly and accurately with success.

Not only is movement time important, but the time required to program a movement response or reaction time can relate directly to the accuracy requirement of the response.[1] This reaction time, which occurs before the motor movement, can depend more on the amplitude of the response or the movement duration, than on task complexity or target size.

Movement responses can be altered by introducing a secondary task, or interference task, which draws attention from the primary goal. For example, if someone is relearning how to put on socks following a stroke and also attempts to carry on a conversation, then the time taken to accomplish the primary task of putting on the socks can be increased. Therapists may want to consider the effect that interference tasks have on the primary task when they are helping someone learn a new skill.

HOW THE INDIVIDUAL CONTROLS AND LEARNS MOVEMENT

Researchers are working towards understanding the control system and the requirements for a person to produce movements. The information processing model suggests that individuals process the information in the environment through the peripheral sensory systems and the central nervous system. They are then able to act on this information. Processing of different pieces of information can occur concurrently (parallel processing), or information can be understood sequentially (serial processing). Both parallel and serial processing can be required to complete a task.

Choice of responses increases the complexity of tasks. Research in this area implies there is a relationship between the amount of information available and the time required to respond to a stimulus. This suggests that reaction time increases with the number of stimulus alternatives. The complexity of the task created by increasing the number of stimulus alternatives will change the individual's response to the task. The ability to respond to a stimulus can also be affected by how difficult the stimulus is to interpret, or by the cognitive abilities of the individual. Hauer et al[2] found that frail elderly people with cognitive difficulties have decreased ability to perform two tasks at once.

The performance of tasks is also influenced by memory. Usually, when a new task is learned, responses are recorded in the long- and short-term memory, and the individual needs to be able to retain these responses long enough for a skill to be produced. Those engaged in rehabilitation programmes are trying to learn relevant skills that they can reproduce over the long term. However, poor memory will affect this learning: for example, if an occupational therapist is helping a child to learn to use a special page turner with the help of an occupational therapist, the learning of the task is *only* useful if it can be remembered and repeated on another day.

Attention

Attention is the capacity to attend to a task and process information about that task. Attention can be identified as a level of arousal, which can be a positive resource if at the right level. However, if arousal is too high or low, it will act as an impairment to motor control. Interference to a task from outside can tax both the individual and the ability to perform the task, and may even prevent completion of the task. This can be avoided if attention can be maintained on the original task and the interference is not of a magnitude or type to cause a problem for the person. Low and high levels of arousal can detract from motor performance; however, an optimum level of arousal, which may vary with the task, can help provide good performance.

Accurate and appropriate sensory input can enhance performance. Feedback and feedforward systems, including the visual and kinaesthetic systems, provide a person with information about performance. Given enough time, they will allow alterations of performance to be made by the person. Feedback requires time, because it provides information so the person can change or complete a task. Very fast ballistic movements do not have time to benefit from the feedback mechanisms that only time can provide.

Functional results are affected by the sensory and perceptual systems. For example, when a person reaches for an object movement speed may cause an increase in overshooting, or reaching past the object. This increase can be explained by considering that the final arm position is not predetermined. The arm position is determined during the activity (not before it) as a result of a feedforward or feedback mechanism.[3]

Another factor that can affect how people learn and control movement is their perception of safety in movement. People who feel unsafe may alter movement parameters. Research by Robinovitch[4] suggests that individuals scale their action to the perceived risk when attempting a given movement. In this research, the perceived risk was not related to the subject's height, weight, or gender, but was weakly correlated with the reaching excursion required. This suggests that a task will be performed within the ability of an individual. For example, someone who is very comfortable with manoeuvring while sitting in a wheelchair will perceive going down a winding, paved trail at a rapid speed as having limited risk, because the person's ability to manage the risk is high. A novice wheelchair user may perceive the task of going down the same path as being too risky or difficult and will not go down it.

MOTOR LEARNING

Motor learning involves a relatively permanent change in motor performance. Motor learning has occurred when a person acquires a physical skill and retains that skill over time. Research in motor learning has focused on determining the attributes of the learning situation and the environment that enhance learning. Researchers have also worked to understand the underlying mechanisms that enable learning to occur. Practice regimes, memory attributes, transfer of learning, and processes of learning can all contribute to the process of learning new tasks, or learning new methods of performing previously learned tasks.

Practice regimes

Practice regimes can be varied. This variation produces different types of learning. A skill can be practised repeatedly with no interruption between trials. This method of practice is called blocked practice. Interfering tasks can be introduced between repetitions of the task practice, and this is called random practice. Blocked practice of a simple task can improve the performance of the task but usually does not contribute to its retention over time.

Random, or distributed, practice might include performing different tasks between trials of the primary task of interest, or practising different tasks within one session. This type of practice frequently interferes with performance improvement within the session, but helps improve retention of the task over time. Random practice of tasks appears to be more beneficial than blocked practice when working with people with delayed retention of tasks.[5] However, while this is evident in simple movements, it is not necessarily observed in more complex tasks in people who have had strokes. This suggests that the level of cognitive effort in which the subject engages can be a factor in retaining motor skills and transferring them to tasks that are similar. Information about the target of a movement, which can be acquired through visual or other sensory input, can influence the outcome of the movement. Researchers have sometimes provided a target for a person to reach, then removed the target and asked the person to reach or move to where they remember the target was. People with cognitive difficulties find it more difficult to remember where the target was. Bennett and Davids[6] suggested that individuals may use different target information, but can achieve comparable final accuracy. The details of the strategies individuals employed differed with the amount of information available to the individuals.

Some tasks are more easily learned using blocked practice, whereas others may be learned through distributed practice. For example, some children need to communicate in writing with a pencil or pen whereas others can use a computer. There are differences in the ease with which children learn these tasks, based on the method of learning that is used with them. The laboratory exercise at the end of the chapter describes methods of learning to type on a computer. Figure 5.3 demonstrates the different postures used by children doing both activities. The reader is invited to look at the different postures required for the two different tasks and consider some of the issues involved in learning to use these methods of communication. Is computer access easily available to people where you live? Do you know what types of adapted access to computers are available?

Explicit and implicit processes

Explicit and implicit processes are thought to mediate skill acquisition. In an explicit process, there is a correspondence between the performer's morphology and the environment, leading to goal attainment. For explicit learning, therapists can tap consciously available processes and instruct the performer about environmental features, task-related feedback, and movement organisation. However, for force generation, which is part of the

Figure 5.3 Writing and using a keyboard.

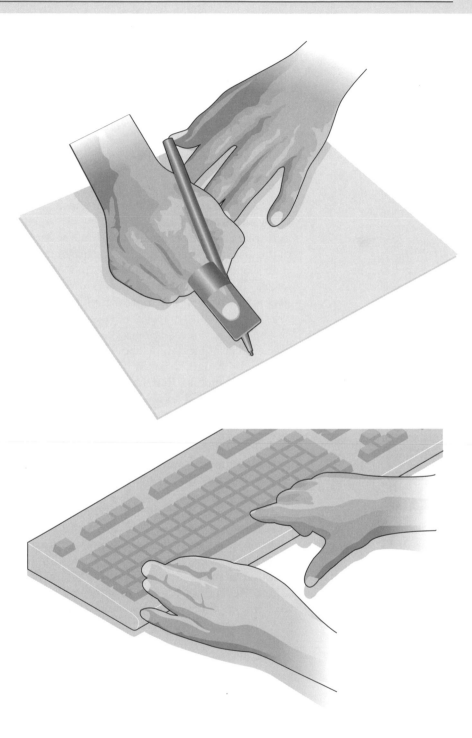

information not readily available to the individual, the therapist can appropriately structure the environment in order to compel appropriate force generation as an indirect consequence of the functional activity.[7] The implicit learning process underlies both force generation and the efficiency of movement. Transfer of learning refers to the ability to learn a new skill and have that learning made easier by having learned a previous, similar skill. Swinnen et al[8] suggest that optimal performance of a coordination pattern during acquisition can also optimise new task performance. For example, a person who has learned to propel a manual chair can have less difficulty learning to play sledge hockey than someone who is unfamiliar with wheelchair propulsion. (Sledge hockey is a sport very similar to ice hockey. The individual sits on a sledge with skate blades attached underneath, which is pushed by the athlete using crampons at the end of two sledge hockey sticks.) Alternatively, knowledge of one activity can inhibit the learning of another skill. For example, a child who is able to walk can have difficulty learning to glide on skates, because the movement pattern is different.

INDIVIDUAL CAPABILITIES AND DIFFERENCES IN MOTOR CONTROL AND MOTOR LEARNING

Characteristics of the learner affect the ability of the person to learn and the ability of the therapist to help teach a new skill. One characteristic of the learner that has been shown to affect the ability to learn is age. At one end of this age continuum, young children are learning many new skills for the first time. They learn how to ride bicycles, tie shoelaces, and develop various other skills that encompass the occupations, such as playing, going to school and self-care, that are the components of their lives. At the other end of the continuum, researchers suggest that older adults control and learn movements somewhat differently from younger subjects.

It is thought that anticipatory strategies (strategies by which an individual can anticipate a required movement) begin as early as the age of 4 years.[9] As motor control develops and improves in children, their dependence on visual control declines, so that smooth and stereotyped kinematic movements can show up by the age of 12 years.[10] A number of problems that can occur in childhood may influence the development of motor control of children. For example, some children with developmental performance delays can have prolonged bursts of electromyographic (muscle) activity compared with their age-matched peers with no delays. This prolonged muscle activity can contribute to their inability to produce fast, accurate, unilateral or one-sided movements. These children appear to have more performance errors and greater time inconsistencies than children with typical motor development. These findings suggest that there are important differences in the way the motor control systems of people with developmental coordination difficulties organise their aiming, bilateral responses.[11]

Children with cerebral palsy adapt their movements to deal with control problems. For example, they tend to compensate for a poor ability to pass under a barrier because of motor control difficulties by controlling their vertical position in space and allowing greater safety margins than do children without such problems.[12]

Our understanding of the motor control function of children with difficulties is also enhanced by considering their physical strength. For example, one researcher demonstrated that children with meningomyelocele have poorer hand function than other children of a similar age.[13] It is possible that this poorer hand function could be due to weakness, although it may also be related to hydrocephalus, lower than average intelligence or cerebral hemispheric pathology. If these children receive more practice time, they show an improvement in acquiring and retaining a new skill, so it appears that their fitness or physical strength does not impact on their performance or learning.

Variability in the timing of movements in older adults is also evident. Older subjects show greater timing variability and initiate movements more slowly when moving towards a specified target than do younger subjects.[14] This research suggests that older subjects' movement control can lack movement planning relative to younger subjects' ability to control movement.

KNOWLEDGE OF RESULTS

Knowledge of results is enhanced feedback of information provided to the individual from an external source. This knowledge is supplied by monitoring equipment or by the therapist and appears to be handled in similar ways in younger and older individuals. There do appear to be age-related differences in accuracy when acquiring and retaining new tasks over time. These differences do not appear to occur on transfer tasks.[15] A transfer task is a task that is similar to the learning task, but not identical. It also appears that, for older adults, summary knowledge of results after a group of trials can facilitate more consistent performance.[16] One study, however, suggests that the ability to grip and lift an object was limited by some older people's reduced availability of tactile information.[17] It is known that sensory information can be reduced in older adults, which can contribute to this finding.

Control of rapid aiming movements decreases in quality for older individuals, which suggests there can be a reduction in movement planning. This reduction results in greater time for feedback during movement execution.[14] Walking is slower in older adults, particularly in people who have vision problems. Even when their vision is poor, older individuals use their vision extensively to control movement.[18,19] Given that movement control can require more visual input as people get older, it is important that visual function is maintained at the highest possible level for older individuals. Research suggests that older individuals can process information in a manner similar to younger individuals but that they do so at a slower speed. When time constraints on a task apply, older individuals can rely more on modes of control in which sensation plays a minimum role, i.e. pre-planning of movements or feedforward control.

The older adult appears to program a response for a central target position in the presence of multiple targets for reach.[20] This programming can provide a dilemma to therapists; they will want to help a person improve performance, but without limiting choices of movement. In quick movements, the question remains: does one put the target in a central position, which would be easier for older adults, or vary its position to encourage older adults to increase their repertoire of responses?

CONDITIONS THAT AFFECT MOTOR CONTROL

Unfortunately, a number of disabilities leading to motor control and learning problems can occur in older individuals. Three such problems, hemiplegia, Parkinson's disease, and cerebellar dysfunction, will be discussed here, citing the literature that can benefit the therapist's strategies when working with individuals who have these problems.

Hemiplegia

Individuals who have sustained a cerebral vascular accident (CVA) exhibit a number of problems. In terms of their motor performance, motor intention disorders can include recurrent perseverations, or repetition of a task in response to subsequent stimulae, and continuous perseverations or abnormal prolongations of a current activity. It appears that these types of perseveration can occur in individuals with either right or left hemisphere damage, except in those people who have sustained right posterior lesions. It appears, then, that there is an interaction between the type of perseveration and the site of the lesion in the brain.[21]

Compared with control individuals, individuals with hemiplegia have movements that appear segmented or less fluid. The movements also demonstrate greater variability and greater deflection from the line of path, when the person is asked to follow a particular line of movement. These individuals also demonstrate difficulty in stabilising the trunk, suggesting that there can be dissociation between the balance control system and finer motor movements. These deficits can be made more problematic because of short-term memory loss.[12] Individuals with left CVAs and apraxia appear to require more trials than other individuals.[22]

Following a CVA, individuals can also have sustained visual distortion. A novel study evaluated the effects of prism adaptations on various neglect symptoms, including left neglect in which people shift their perception of where the midline is to the right of where it truly is. All the people who were exposed to the optical shift of the visual field improved their manual body line demonstration, and this effect lasted at least 2 hours after the removal of the prism.[23] Another researcher, evaluating visual inattention, or having a blind field, suggested that not only orientation, but also the curve structure and ordering of letters are registered non-consciously in the blind field.[24] The findings of this author suggested that shape is much better perceived in blind sight than was previously thought, and this is independent of motor control. This implies that the main deficit in this problem is one of consciousness, and loss of unconscious vision is far from total. There can be a strong link between visual consciousness, attention, and object perception.[24]

Different lesions have been found to affect motor control in different ways. Researchers have suggested that people who have frontal lesions can control simple movements when the movement requirements are presented in novel conditions. This does not appear to affect the rate of acquiring new skills. The frontal cortex can be more important than the aspects of learning that require sensory-motor function,[25] for closed-loop motor control.

Therapists are able to enhance control and learning in older adults, fashioning the learning experience by accommodating known limitations that are encountered in the older adult, as described in the literature.[26]

There is evidence that random practice is more effective than blocked practice, with respect to retention over time, for hemiparetic patients attempting to learn motor skills.[5] However, this is in contrast to work by Tse,[27] which did not find a difference for people with hemiplegia when an interference task was included between trials of a new motor task.

Rushworth et al[28] argued that deficits of the left hemisphere are explained as an impairment of response selection, and are not just a sequencing problem. It appears that people with left hemiplegia are more impaired on a demanding task of discrimination learning, that imposes a greater memory load but does not have a response selection element. Results of another study demonstrate the need to control cognitive task demands when exploring the motor capabilities of individuals with left brain damage.[29] There appears also to be a distinction, in individuals with neglect, between visual processing used for object recognition and visual processing used to guide action. Research has demonstrated that people show an increased level of grip force for objects presented in their left-hemi-field, which supports the finding that there is a difference between visual processing used for object recognition and visual processing used to guide action.[30] These findings, when pooled together, give us an indication that individuals who have sustained a CVA have very complex difficulties. Therapists who work with these individuals know that the problems are complex.

The studies mentioned above provide us with an insight into some of these complexities and give us opportunities to attempt methods of teaching that can contribute to learning for these individuals. For example, therapists can be encouraged to further a person's motor learning if they know that despite the fact that object recognition is not possible in the early stages of hemiplegic neglect, movement characteristics can still be possible using that side. The study on prisms[23] gives us a new way of considering methods of rehabilitation with people who have hemi-inattention or neglect. The student or therapist reading this may want to consider alternative ways of providing therapy, structure and feedback to make use of those characteristics which are inherent in the individual with hemiplegia. As Masjak says, 'It is proposed that only through the combination of clinical research and critical introspection of our treatment practices can we gain better insight into the motor learning behaviours of stroke patients.'[31]

Parkinson's disease

Another group upon whom much attention has been focused by researchers trying to understand human movement and ameliorate movement problems, are those who have Parkinson's disease. It has been suggested that individuals with Parkinson's disease do not differ from the rest of us in their methods of processing motor adaptation and motor skill learning.[32] However, it has also been suggested that they can improve their performance on new tasks but are dependent on augmented information.

If a task is closed-loop (i.e. a task that occurs in a predictable environment and where the task is similar each time it occurs), it can be accompanied by speed reduction to ensure accuracy (an example of Fitt's law).[33] Another study supports this slowing of movement. The authors suggest that individuals with Parkinson's disease have been observed to increase their movement time, pause more between tasks, and have jerky movements when a secondary task comprises a motor component.[34] Despite the fact that both speed and movement appear to decrease in people with Parkinson's disease, some work[35] demonstrates an ability to increase speed in single ballistic, or very quick, movements that are so speedy that feedback is not possible. In aiming movements like these, people with Parkinson's disease may be able to show improvement, and there can be the possibility of decreasing bradykinesia (slowed movement) by training. Other work[36] also demonstrates that there seems to be a deficit in motor functioning when two separate motor programs are superimposed in individuals with Parkinson's disease.

Cerebellar dysfunction

Decreased cerebellar function, or lesions in this area, can have a strong impact on functional ability in individuals. After therapy these individuals can perform almost normally in skills that entail slow movement, but in fast movements their performance doesn't appear to improve to this extent. The consequences of cerebellar dysfunction are also evident in the time needed to initiate simulated behaviours[37] when an individual is required to execute a volitional movement. As therapists who work with individuals with cerebellar dysfunction or Parkinson's disease know, there is a deficit in motor functioning. The importance of this research in these areas of functioning is that it suggests that some of these lost skills can be relearned.

It becomes apparent that individuals with neurological impairment or damage must relearn old skills or learn new skills.[38] They can do this learning using slightly different methods from individuals who do not have neurological problems.

ENABLING MOTOR LEARNING: INSTRUCTION BY THERAPISTS

Researchers have looked at the characteristics of instructions that are provided to enhance learning.[39,40] Instruction can be provided by verbally describing the task, modelling or demonstrating the task, providing visual examination of expert models (perhaps showing illustrations, videos, or CD ROM images of experts), and motivating the learner. An instructor can also structure practice, using blocked or random practice.

Knowledge of results can enhance learning, if it is used effectively. Knowledge of results could be provided by videotaping or measuring response time. It could also be given as verbal information provided by the therapist. If knowledge of results is very well described and discrete, then motor performance can be improved.[40] Isokinetic torque production has been noted to be greater and more reliable when visual feedback is given to the individual than when there has been no visual feedback.[39] However, visual feedback will not be as advantageous once a skill has been learned.[40] Knowledge of results can have both immediate and persistent influences on learning.

Mental practice or mental imagery is the mental rehearsal of a cognitive skill without actually producing the skill. For example, an individual can mentally go through an activity prior to performing it. It has been suggested that this mental practice or imagery can enhance movement characteristics. Imagery training can allow individuals to improve motor performance as measured by speed. It has been suggested that mental imagery can improve the acquisition of spatial–temporal patterns of movement, and that there are different processes in mental imagery and motor or movement imagery of the practised task.[41]

Imagery training by itself can provide an important approach to movement and may result in a significant shift of peak velocity towards a target. This suggests that using motor imagery can improve trajectories of movement and that visual and motor imagery involve different processes. However, this work has not been conducted on individuals who have movement difficulties and the caveat remains that it may not apply to people with movement difficulties. Therapists can attempt imagery training to see if it will be effective in an individual with whom they are working, but research has not been conducted to assure its accuracy.

There is a definite sense amongst therapists that providing an activity with a purpose that is understood or chosen by the individual, will improve the performance of the activity and the functioning of the skill. These activities, purposes, and skills can then be pooled into occupations. Ferguson and Trombly[42] found that added-purpose occupation resulted in increased motor learning compared with non-added-purpose occupation. This suggests that added purpose can enhance a more permanent aspect of performance, or motor learning. Ma and Trombly's account[43] of the effect of occupational therapy on an individual with a stroke found that using meaningful goal objects improved coordinated movement.

It is suggested that rehabilitation goals are limited if physical parameters are the only outcomes required. Therapists should use functional activities because they cognitively challenge individuals, help them gain skills more quickly, and seem to help them retain skills longer. If the ultimate goal of therapy is to enhance individuals' abilities to perform occupational tasks that are important to them, these techniques can transfer to everyday life.[44]

Lin et al[45] compared and evaluated the movements of people ringing a bell in what they called 'natural conditions' (when the bell would ring) and in 'impoverished conditions' (when the bell would fail to ring). Better quality reaching movements were elicited in the natural conditions than in the impoverished conditions. This suggests that including normal outputs in activities will elicit better movement. Although this work was conducted with people who had no movement difficulties, it may be of value to a therapist to try to use activities that have a natural outcome. The manipulation of functional goals may enhance the motor performance of persons with disabilities. Added-purpose can enhance the longer-lasting aspect of performance – that of motor learning.[42]

Newell and Valvano[46] suggest that the challenge for the therapist is to select information constraints that can induce effective and efficient strategies for task-related qualitative and quantitative changes. A further challenge is to ensure that these changes result in functional output in the movement dynamics which are important for the individual.

SUMMARY

This chapter suggests that therapy is not a passive process for the therapist or the learner. Current knowledge about how people who have physical difficulties learn is far from complete, but the therapist can draw on a body of knowledge about how new skills are learned.

In fact, research into the therapeutic use of theories of motor control and motor learning is only beginning, although some excellent work has already been done. Therapists have at their disposal various technical practice regimes, such as sensory feedback, as well as current knowledge about motor control and motor learning processes. However, since most of the research into motor control and motor learning has been with people who do not have physical problems, therapists need to be aware that they are applying this information to a group of people not included in the original research. Therefore therapists should be vigilant in observing the effects of using these techniques, and should try to keep up with current literature on using motor control and motor learning principles effectively. Therapists should be engaged in observing, measuring and recording treatment outcomes, such as the speed and accuracy with which new tasks are carried out. In this way, understanding of motor control and motor learning in the individuals with whom they work can be used to change and improve therapy techniques.

QUESTIONS BASED ON THE CASE

1. Put yourself in the position of Ms Spiegel's occupational therapist. Decide if you need more information about the disability that Ms Spiegel has acquired.
2. Describe the physical problems that Ms Spiegel has. Explain how these problems will affect her rehabilitation.
3. List possible occupational difficulties that Ms Spiegel will encounter. The overall difficulties are evident in the case, but can you think in more detail about some of the problems that will be encountered by someone in Ms Spiegel's position?
4. Choose two skills that Ms Spiegel will want to relearn. Identify the characteristics of the skills you have chosen. For example, are the skills open or closed? Are they discrete or continuous? Think about all the characteristics of skills described in this chapter and apply them to the skills you have chosen to consider. Describe the steps or components required to perform the skills.
5. Explain the methods you would use to teach the skills using the principles of motor learning.

continued overpage

6. The occupational therapist will use knowledge of results. What type of knowledge of results might she use? Why might this be helpful?
7. Describe the difficulties that you and Ms Spiegel might encounter as she relearns these skills. Use the knowledge you have gained concerning the specific problems someone who has had a stroke might encounter when learning a new skill.
8. Teach one of the skills that you have chosen to one of your friends or classmates. Which of the methods that you used were successful? Which methods did your learner think were most helpful?
9. Although this question is not directly related to the information in this chapter, it is important to consider. Do you think that Ms Spiegel will be able to return to her former occupation? What do you think she should do?

Laboratory Exercise: Learning and Teaching One-Handed Typing

One of the issues that Ms Spiegel, herself considers important is learning to use a computer again. It does not appear that using a computer mouse will be difficult with her left hand, but learning to type with one hand will need some teaching and practice.

This exercise uses the skill of teaching a sequence of keyboard letters starting from the home row key positions for the left hand. This will provide the reader with the opportunity to learn about whole versus part teaching and to see how effective each method might be for this task. In whole teaching, the entire skill is taught and practised at once, whereas in progressive part teaching, part of the task is taught, then extra parts are added to the initial part. Skills that are simple can be taught using the whole teaching method, but as the skills become more complex, it is difficult to remember the whole skill and part teaching is more appropriate.

Method

Work in pairs for this exercise.

One person in the pair will learn the key sequence for the left hand, using the whole method; the other person will use the progressive part method.

Consider the home keys for the left hand to be J, H, G and F. This is usually the standard used by therapists when teaching one-handed typing.

The sequence of keys that you will be asked to learn (without looking at the keyboard during the retention task) is: J, T, N, R, H, I, V, Y.

Whole learning technique

The individuals using the whole learning technique will practice the entire sequence 30 times, using a cue card (which you create) and looking at the keys. Every 5th practice, determine how long it takes to type the sequence, starting with the 10th trial (10th, 15th, 20th, 25th and 30th). Have your partner use a stopwatch or a second hand on a watch to determine how long it takes you to do the task.

Wait 10 minutes.

Type the sequence without looking at the cue card or the keys. Have your partner time two trials. Record the number of errors and the time required to complete the task.

Progressive part technique

The individuals using progressive part learning will practise the sequence in the following way.

In trials 1 through 5 type the letters J T.

In trials 6 through 10 type J T N R.

In trials 11 through 15 type J T N R H I

In trials 16 through 30 type J T N R H I V Y.

Have your partner time the 20th, 25th and 30th trials.

Wait 10 minutes, and then have your partner time two trials without you looking at a cue card or the keyboard. Record the number of errors and the time required to complete the task.

Note that this may be a useful method of teaching one-handed typing to people who might have to type with only one hand because of a stroke, cerebral palsy, upper extremity amputation or other disability.

Questions

Compare the two groups.

Which group was faster at the 20th, 25th and 30th trials? Compare the differences between the two groups at each performance of the whole sequence. Describe the differences at each of the trial times.

Was there a difference between groups on the retention trial? Were these differences timing or error differences (remember Fitt's Law – did you sacrifice speed for accuracy or vice versa)?

Describe another motor skill you could teach to someone who has sustained a CVA and discuss how and why you would have this individual practise this skill, in terms of a whole versus part method of practice. Teach this skill to your partner, using some of the techniques described in this chapter.

Describe how knowledge about whole versus part learning might help you design practice sessions when teaching new tasks to individuals.

REFERENCES

1. Lajoie JM, Franks JM. The control of rapid aiming movements – variations in response accuracy and complexity. Acta Psychol 1997; 97(3):289–305.
2. Hauer K, Marburger C, Oster P. Motor performance deteriorates with simultaneously performed cognitive tasks in geriatric patients. Arch Phys Med Rehabil 2002; 83(2):217–223.
3. Adamovich SV, Berkinblit MB, Fookson O, Poizner H. Pointing in 3D space to remembered targets. II. Effects of movement speed toward kinesthetically defined targets. Exp Brain Res 1999; 125(2):200–210.
4. Robinovitch SN. Perception of postural limits during reaching. J Mot Behav 1998; 30(4):352–358.

5. Hanlon RE. Motor learning following unilateral stroke. Arch Phys Med Rehabil 1996; 77(8):811–815.
6. Bennett S, Davids K. Manipulating peripheral visual information in manual aiming – explaining the notion of specificity of learning. Hum Mov Sci 1998; 17(2):261–287.
7. Gentile AM. Implicit and explicit processes during acquisition of functional skills. Scand J Occup Ther 1998; 5(1):7–16.
8. Swinnen SP, Lee TD, Verschueren SM, et al. Interlimb coordination – learning and transfer under different feedback conditions. Hum Mov Sci 1997; 16(6):749–785.
9. Pare M, Dugas C. Developmental changes in prehension during childhood. Exp Brain Res 1999; 125(3):239–247.
10. Kuhtz-Buschbeck JP, Stolze H, Johnk K, et al. Development of prehension movements in children: a kinematic study. Exp Brain Res 1998; 122(4):424–432.
11. Huh J, Williams HG, Burke JR. Development of bilateral motor control in children with developmental coordination disorders. Dev Med Child Neurol 1998; 40(7):474–484.
12. Vandermeer ALH. Visual guidance of passing under a barrier. Early Develop Parent 1997; 6(3–4):149–157.
13. Muen WJ, Bannister CM. Hand function in subjects with spina bifida. Eur J Pediatri Surg 1997; 7 (Suppl): 118–122.
14. Yan JH, Thomas JR, Stelmach GE. Aging and rapid aiming arm movement control. Exp Aging Res 1998; 24(2):155–168.
15. Wishart LR, Lee TD. Effects of aging and reduced relative frequency of knowledge of results on learning a motor skill. Percept Mot Skills 1997; 84(3 Pt 1):1107–1122.
16. Carnahan H, Vandervoort AA, Swanson LR. The influence of summary knowledge of results and aging on motor learning. Res Q Exerc Sport 1996; 67(3):280–287.
17. Cole KJ, Rotella DL, Harper JG. Tactile impairments cannot explain the effect of age on a grasp and lift task. Exp Brain Res 1998; 121(3):263–269.
18. Spaulding S, Patla AE, Rietdyk S, et al. Gait characteristics during dark and light adaptation in individuals with age-related maculopathy. Gait Posture 1995; 3(4):227–235.
19. Elliott DB, Patla AE, Flanagan JG, et al. The Waterloo vision and mobility study: postural control strategies in subjects with ARM. Ophthalmic Physiol Opt 1995; 15(6):553–559.
20. Chaput S, Proteau L. Aging and motor control. J Gerontol Series B – Psychological Sciences and Social Sciences 1996; 51(6):346–355.
21. Annoni G, Pegna A, Michel C, et al. Motor perseverations: a function of the side and the site of a cerebral lesion. Eur Neurol 1998; 40(2):84–90.
22. Poole JL. Application of motor learning principles in occupational therapy. Am J Occup Ther 1991; 45(6):531–537.
23. Rossetti Y, Rode G, Pisella L, et al. Prism adaptation to a rightward optical deviation rehabilitates left hemispatial neglect. Nature 1998; 395(6698):166–169.
24. Marcel AJ. Blindsight and shape perception: deficit of visual consciousness or of visual function? Brain 1998; 121(8):1565–1588.
25. Chouinard MJ, Rouleau I, Richer F. Closed-loop sensorimotor control and acquisition after lesions. Brain Cogn 1998; 37(1):178–182.
26. Porter J. Motor learning in the older adult. Issues Aging 1996; 19(1):14–17.
27. Tse DW. Practice conditions and motor learning in individuals post stroke: a pilot-study comparing random and block practice. [Thesis. The University of Western Ontario.] 1998.
28. Rushworth MF, Nixon PD, Wade DT, et al. The left hemisphere and the selection of learned actions. Neuropsychologia 1998; 36(1):11–24.
29. Spatt J, Goldenberg G. Speed of motor execution and apraxia. J Clin Exp Neuropsychol 1997; 19(6):850–856.
30. Shaw A, Jackson SR, Harvey M, et al. Grip force scaling after hemispatial neglect. NeuroReport 1997; 8(17):3837–3840.
31. Majenk MJ. Application of motor learning principles to the stroke population. Top Stroke Rehabil 1996; 3(2):27–59.
32. Agostino R, Sanes JN, Hallett M. Motor skill learning in Parkinson's disease. J Neurol Sci 1996; 139(2):218–226.

33. Verschueren SM, Swinnen SP, Dom R, De Weerdt W. Interlimb coordination in patients with Parkinson's disease: motor learning deficits and the importance of augmented information feedback. Exp Brain Res 1997; 113(3):497–508.
34. Vangemmert AWA, Teulings HL, Stelmach GE. The influence of mental and motor load on handwriting movements in Parkinsonian patients. Acta Psychol 1998; 100(1–2):161–175.
35. Platz T, Brown RG, Marsden CD. Training improves the speed of aimed movements in Parkinson's disease. Brain 1998; 121(Pt 3):505–514.
36. Suri RE, Albani C, Glattfelder AH. Analysis of double-joint movements in controls and in Parkinsonian patients. Exp Brain Res 1998; 118(2):243–250.
37. Topka H, Massaquoi SG, Benda N, Hallett M. Motor learning in patients with cerebellar degeneration. J Neurol Sci 1998; 158(2):164–172.
38. Hochstenbach J, Mulder T. Neuropsychology and the relearning of motor skills following stroke. Int J Rehabil Res 1999; 22(1):11–19.
39. Kim HJ, Kramer JF. Effectiveness of visual feedback during isokinetic exercise. J Orthop Sports Phys Ther 1997; 26(6):318–323.
40. Salmoni AW, Schmidt RA, Walter CB. Knowledge of results and motor learning: a review and reappraisal. Psychological Bulletin 1984; 95:355–386.
41. Yaguez L, Nagel D, Hoffman H, et al. A mental route to motor learning: improving trajectorial kinematics through imagery training. Behav Brain Res 1998; 90(1):95–106.
42. Ferguson JM, Trombly CA. The effect of added-purpose and meaningful occupation on motor learning. Am J Occup Ther 1997; 51(7):508–515.
43. Ma HI, Trombly CA. A synthesis of the effects of occupational therapy for persons with stroke, part II: remediation of impairments. Am J Occup Ther 2002; 56(3):260–274.
44. Stevans J, Hall KG. Motor skill acquisition strategies for rehabilitation of low back pain. J Orthop Sports Phys Ther 1998; 28(3):165–167.
45. Lin KC, Wu CY, Trombly CA. Effects of task goal on movement kinematics and line bisection performance in adults without disabilities. Am J Occup Ther 1998; 52(3):179–187.
46. Newell KM, Valvano J. Therapeutic intervention as a constraint in learning and relearning movement skills. Scand J Occup Ther 1998; 5(2):51–57.

SECTION 2

Applications in occupational therapy

SECTION CONTENTS

Chapter 6

Balance: adequate balance is the basis for occupation

CHAPTER CONTENTS

To engage in any occupation, good balance is required. Without good balance in standing, sitting or kneeling positions, people can be so preoccupied with trying to stop themselves from falling over that they are unable to do anything. A discussion of balance requires consideration of biomechanics and motor control because balance is a phenomenon needing many mechanical principles to explain it. Balance also requires control by the person. Although balance seems like a simple task, it is actually very complex and not easy to achieve once it has been hampered by physical problems.

Occupational therapists often work with people who need controlled balance as an underpinning for their occupations. Many activities are difficult to perform without a stable balance state. Balance control includes balance during sitting, standing or moving from place to place during occupational tasks.

It is frequently the case that balance must be assessed and treated so individuals can fully and safely engage in activities. Prior to assessing balance, the occupational therapist needs an understanding of many balance mechanisms, including aspects of the physical and sensory systems influencing balance. Therapists also need to understand the risks that can precipitate the occurrence of a slip or trip. Therapists work towards helping to prevent falls from occurring, and then encourage people to be engaged in the activities of their choice.

An understanding of balance mechanisms includes being familiar with both the mechanical characteristics and some of the visual and spatial orientation characteristics that have been found to play a major role in posture and balance. For example, some visual characteristics, such as vertical lines on a wall, can help balance, whereas flat light, such as occurs on a grey day when the sun is not shining, decreases cues in the environment that help balance.

In this chapter some of the problems of balance in individuals with particular problems are explained. Factors in the environment are described. Assessments of trips and falls, from both clinical and biomechanical perspectives, are examined. How people respond to perturbations is discussed, along with methods for preventing trips or falls.

Read the following case. There will be questions about it, related to balance, at the end of the chapter.

CASE STUDY: MS JENNIFER HENDERSON

Ms Jennifer Henderson is a 25-year-old woman who sustained a serious traumatic brain injury (TBI) when she was driving home from a party one night. She caused a major accident in which she was seriously injured; her friend Connie, whom she was driving home, was also hurt and had to have her dominant right arm amputated. Ms Henderson was charged by the police for causing an accident. It is uncertain how the legal proceedings will go because she is still far from even understanding what happened to her and her friend. She also has no money to pay for legal assistance and this will need to be provided by the courts.

She lived in a small apartment building in her town with her friend, Susan. They shared the rent and some of the upkeep of the apartment together. They spent time together, going to parties on the weekends, watching television and going to movies.

Her parents also live in the small town. They want to support their daughter, but they have no understanding of what her head injury means. They expect she will be better soon and do not understand that she may not regain all the abilities she had before her accident.

The setting

Ms Henderson was returned to the town where she lives after she had been medically stabilised following her head injury. She has many problems, including a labile affect, physical aggression and minimal problem-solving skills. She is presently in a long-term care facility with people who are over the age of 70 years. She could not cope in a family setting or on her own. She needs to be watched during the day because of her challenging behaviour, but seems to be fine at night. There is no other place, such as a rehabilitation hospital or unit, for her to go to in her town.

Occupational therapy student

Ms Andrews is an occupational therapy student who has successfully finished all her academic course work and is now in her final clinical placement. She is in the third week of her placement in the long-term care facility. She is under the supervision of Ms Gwen O'Keefe, who has experience in working with older people but has little experience with people as young as Ms Henderson, nor is she very familiar with what can be expected during Ms Henderson's stay in the facility.

The individual

Ms Henderson is a 25-year-old woman who incurred the TBI during a motor vehicle accident 6 months ago. She progressed slowly during her hospitalisation immediately following the accident and took 2 months to come out of a coma. She is in a long-term care facility primarily because of her behaviour but also because she has many physical problems.

Ms Henderson was unemployed at the time of the accident. She had left school at the age of 16 and had worked in a small store and in a bar in town, but she had not held down a job for more than 6 months at any one place.

Physical abilities

Ms Henderson has limited physical abilities. She can sit up without support in a wheelchair. She can stand without assistance, but her balance is not good enough for her to engage in any occupations, because she is likely to fall. When the therapist pushes her slightly from behind, she will fall if there isn't someone there to support her, so she does not have normal responses to perturbations. She does not have strategies to stop herself from falling:

she does not put a foot forward if she is pushed from behind, and she does not put her hands out to avert a fall.

She can walk with a walker, but it is awkward for her. She is strong enough to walk through the halls of the facility, but has difficulty with surfaces that are more uneven, for example the path outside the centre. Because she uses a walker, she cannot use her arms for any other activity or to hold anything while she is walking.

Her arm function is reasonable in that she can carry out some gross motor tasks and has enough dexterity to dress herself while she is sitting down. She can do some work in the kitchen, again while she is seated, but she has difficulty concentrating.

Emotional status

It is difficult to know what Ms Henderson is feeling about her head injury. Her acting out and anger could be either a response to the injury or a result of it. Whatever the cause of her emotions, they need to be dealt with by the people who work with her, her family and her friends. She has almost no ability to control her anger, which can be expressed at the least frustration. She has very little insight into her emotions or into the consequences of the head injury. Her emotional state makes it difficult to work with her.

EXPLORING ISSUES WITH MS HENDERSON

It is difficult to explore issues with Ms Henderson because of her head injury and her minimal comprehension of what the injury will mean for her in the long term. It is also challenging to look at long-term issues because the therapist cannot be sure how much of a recovery Ms Henderson will make.

Ms Henderson is able to articulate some of her wants, despite her inability to understand fully what is happening to her. She has two big desires, but has little understanding of why she is unable to fulfil them right now and what it may take to get her to them. She wants to go home. She wants to be able to do things in her apartment, the way she used to do them. She also wants to return to her social life and spend time partying with her friends.

Ms O'Keefe is not sure what is in store, long term, for Ms Henderson. She is not sure if she will be able to leave the long-term facility and return to apartment living. She knows Ms Henderson is unemployed so she must seek funding from wherever she can to help her get equipment and support. Ms O'Keefe has had to do a great deal of reading about head injuries and she has been in touch with therapists in neighbouring communities who are more knowledgeable than she is about problems related to head injuries. She also knows that Ms Henderson may have to face charges related to the accident, so future plans are difficult to make.

Ms O'Keefe has been able to establish a rapport with Ms Henderson and is helping her to focus a bit more on the problems that she faces at the moment, such as her very poor balance which makes it difficult for her to do anything while she is standing up.

Think about Ms Henderson as you go through this chapter. Some of her problems are indeed hard to solve, but you should be able to come up with some ideas for therapy that will be meaningful for her.

FUNDAMENTAL CONCEPTS FOR UNDERSTANDING POSTURE AND BALANCE

- *Balance control*: This is when a person is able to maintain or control balance during sitting, standing or moving from place to place during occupational tasks.
- *Balance mechanisms*: These are the mechanical characteristics and some of the visual and spatial orientation parameters that have been found to play a major role in posture and balance.
- *Base of support*: This is the area under the mass (we can usually think of it as the area under a person's body), which supports the mass or person from falling. The base of support for someone who is standing would be the area between and under the feet. The base of support for someone who uses a walker would be the area surrounded by the walker legs and the person's feet.
- *Centre of mass*: This is the point about which all the body mass is balanced. The centre of mass of an object of uniform shape and density, such as a rubber ball, would be the centre of the ball. The centre of mass of a standing person is somewhere in the trunk of the body.
- *Dynamic balance*: This is balance while movement occurs. A person can be considered to have dynamic balance while moving but staying upright.
- *Static balance*: Balance occurs when a person is not moving, such as when a person is standing very still.
- *Visual anchors*: The person focuses on a specific point after movement, to enhance balance control. For example, a skater can focus on a particular point in an arena after spinning, in order to enhance the probability of maintaining balance.
- *Visual surround:* This is the visual characteristics or appearance of the environment.

MECHANISMS OF BALANCE

Balance is considered to be maintained when the centre of mass is over the base of support. The centre of mass is the centre point in the body or body segment, at which all the mass is theoretically present. In an upright human, the centre of mass is somewhere within the chest area. The exact location of the centre of mass depends on the individual's body size and the distribution of various tissues, such as muscle and bone, that have different densities. For example, if Ms Henderson is stooped over because of physical problems related to her injury, her centre of mass will not be in the usual position, but will be forward relative to her base of support. The base of support must be under the centre of mass to provide stability.

In standing, the base of support is the area including the two feet and the space between the feet. If a person is standing using a walker, the base of support is expanded to include the feet, the area between the feet and the area from the feet to the edges of the walker. Because the base of support has enlarged, the person now has a safer area within which to balance. In sitting, the base of support is the area which is in contact with the seating surface.

Maintenance of standing balance following small pushes, changes in position, or perturbations is thought to be controlled primarily by the muscles around the ankles. Ms Henderson is having difficulties, because she cannot maintain balance while doing another activity, such as reaching into a cupboard. Larger perturbations require muscles at the hip joint to return a person to an upright position, and very large perturbations require a person to take a step in order to prevent loss of balance.[1]

Proprioceptive information from the ankle and the neck muscles is used for two tasks: balance control and orientation of the body in space; and for the integration of both these tasks.[2] If this sensory input is impaired, as may occur after a person has had a stroke or a traumatic brain injury such as that experienced by Ms Henderson, balance may be impaired. Balance impairment can occur even if a person has good muscle function.

Balance can be broken down into static balance and dynamic balance. Static balance occurs when no movement is happening. This does not mean the muscles are inactive. It means only that the person is not moving or, more likely, moving so little it is difficult to see the movement. For example, consider a child with cerebral palsy sitting in a chair. While the child is sitting in the chair, balance can be maintained by supporting the child's forearms on the arms of the chair. The child will probably not fall over, because of the support, which prevents the child from leaning too far over to the side or from slipping down from the chair seat. Although perhaps the child's arms are unable to be used in a functional manner, with the provision of an adequate seating system to appropriately support the trunk, the child's arms can be freed to participate in an activity. Sitting static balance is still being maintained, but by adding supports to establish sitting balance, function with the upper extremities is also possible.

On observation, static balance seems to consist of no movement, but there are extensive requirements for balance to be maintained. The muscles are often functioning to maintain balance. 'Balance is not based on a fixed set of equilibrium reflexes but on a flexible, functional motor skill that can adapt with training and experience.'[3] Recent research has supported the concept of a postural control network for standing balance recovery, as opposed to control through a feedback reflex loop.[4] Vision and orientation in space are also important for balance.[4] A person must either have good vision, or be able to compensate with other senses. Many postural adjustments are chosen well before the sensory information characterising the nature of the object is available.[5]

Dynamic balance, in contrast with static balance, occurs during movement. Figure 6.1 provides an example of dynamic balance. Can you think of another example of when dynamic balance is essential in keeping a person upright? Dynamic balance can be affected by various characteristics of the person. For example, walking is a type of dynamic balance. Balance

Figure 6.1 Girl going downhill on a scooter.

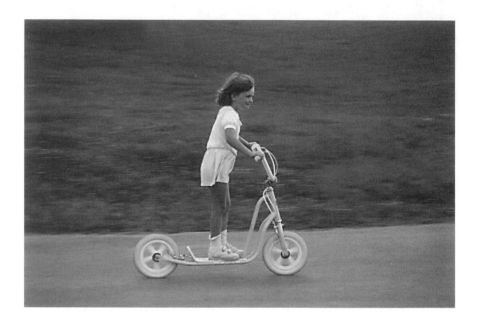

can be affected by changes in the timing of arm swinging.[6] One can imagine that a person who has had a stroke with one of the arms affected may be hindered from good walking balance because of the poor arm function, as well as any difficulty with the leg. Small children have been observed to adapt to environmental changes with changes in gait.[7] An individual with Parkinson's disease who walks in a shopping mall with a wheeled walker is in a state of dynamic balance. As the person moves, the centre of mass is maintained over the base of support that includes both the person's feet and the walker legs. This dynamic balance will be maintained as long as the person is moving and does not fall. Some research[8] suggests that people with Parkinson's disease can adapt to changes in the environment. This finding may help therapists to encourage people with Parkinson's disease to attempt tasks under varying environmental conditions.

It has been argued that moving to standing from sitting is the most frequently performed component of activities of daily living.[9] Standing-from-sitting is another dynamic balance activity that requires complex interactions of the muscles and sensory systems to prevent a fall from occurring. Momentum, a biomechanical term, is the product of the mass of a body and its velocity, and plays an important role in the task of rising from a seated position.[10] If there is a large momentum, because either the person is heavy or is moving quickly, it can be more difficult for the person to maintain and control balance while rising to standing. Moving from lying to sitting can also be difficult and it has been found that tasks requiring trunk flexion and arm use are the most difficult for frail elderly individuals. Alexander et al suggested that improvement in this activity might be enhanced by working on trunk movements and arm strengthening.[11] Sitting balance, as measured by the Functional Independence Measure[12], has also been shown to have an impact on the rehabilitation of individuals following brain injury.

Dynamic balance is often a prerequisite for functional activities. It is difficult for a person who is unable to prevent a fall during movement to perform occupational tasks. In order for the individual to complete a task successfully, balance control and the orientation of the body need to be integrated with the task.[2]

Age-related balance issues

Age-related changes affect balance function, resulting in poorer balance in older individuals than in younger people. Researchers have addressed the conditions under which balance is compromised in the elderly.[13–16] There can be increases in the time muscles take to start contracting and disruptions in typical patterns of muscle timing in older people when there is a threat to balance.[1,17] Older individuals can also have more difficulties when sensory inputs are reduced.[1] Different reflex control strategies have been noted to be invoked more readily in the elderly than in younger people.[15]

Aging can lead to a decrease in the detection of events that are occurring and in responding to and controlling postural sway.[14] Some researchers imply that although older adults require more time to make a voluntary step, they move as quickly as younger people in an involuntary situation (in which they may not have control of the inputs to encourage normal postural movement). This implies an underestimate of the ability of healthy elderly adults to respond when their balance becomes destabilized.[18]

Changing stable visual anchors (points a person can focus on, to help maintain balance), combining a task with a requirement for cognitive activity, or presence of low light intensity (such as is found inside an elevator) can have negative effects on postural stability in older people.[19] The ability to recover from an external push or perturbation appears to require greater attention in older adults than in younger adults. This implies that there will be an increased risk of balance loss if attention is not allocated to postural recovery.[13,20]

Some authors have evaluated strategies to improve balance in elderly people. Postural sway has been noted to be better in older women who do brisk walking than in people in a control group,[21] and present activity level, as opposed to former athletic performance, demonstrates protection for postural balance.[22] During normal lighting conditions, as opposed to dim or dark situations, people are able to balance more readily.[23]

Balance in the presence of physical difficulties

Pathology can result in difficulties with posture and balance. For example, people with Parkinson's disease can have difficulty responding to support or different ground conditions under their feet. They may have a gait pattern that causes their centre of mass to move forward and out of their base of support. Those individuals who have Alzheimer's disease without extrapyramidal signs have no difficulty changing their postural set in response to support condition changes.[24] People with Alzheimer dementia, however, have decreased ability to suppress visual input when it is incongruent with the situation in which they are trying to maintain balance.[24] Individuals who have experienced strokes have been evaluated for their ability to control the trunk while doing a reaching movement. It appears that people who have had a stroke have difficulty with smooth trunk movements during reaching.[25] This finding may have some implications for the balance ability of people who have had strokes.

Evaluating safety margins or the area within the base of support where the person can safely move the centre of mass, can be used as a control strategy to prevent falls.[26] An individual prone to falls may not know how to reach or sway without causing a fall. Some older individuals may lack awareness of declines in stability borders, resulting in a tendency to plan movements which can result in a loss of balance.[27]

Strategies to maintain balance

Proprioceptive and vestibular inputs can lead to balance corrections and the interactions of these inputs can vary across muscles depending on the availability of sensory information. If information is not available from one system, it can be obtained from another. Allum and Honegger[28] implied that trunk inputs might be ideal for triggering balance corrections when other inputs, such as input from the vestibular system, or from the ankle or knee, are absent. Children with cerebral palsy sometimes need ankle–foot orthoses to correct ankle function. Static ankle–foot orthoses for these children do not have as positive an effect on balance as do dynamic ankle–foot orthoses.[29]

If they stumble or trip, elderly individuals need to use a longer response time and use their arms to regain balance, however, they appear to use a shorter stride length following a trip. They can move more slowly, to encourage safe movement and maintenance of balance. Older individuals exercise conservative balance control.[17] This implies older people may not move as far to the edges of their base of support, because of concern for safety.

Many different factors can negatively affect balance control. Medications can adversely affect balance, and spectacles that do not have a current prescription also cause problems. The therapist must be aware of these issues.

FACTORS THAT CAN PRECIPITATE A TRIP OR A FALL

Factors related to the physical environment, the person or the occupation in which the person is engaged can precipitate a trip or fall. Therapists can evaluate all three factors and make recommendations to reduce the chances of a trip or fall occurring. They can also help a person make adjustments to the surrounding environment, as well as helping the person be as physically ready as possible. Occupations can also be adapted in conjunction with the wishes of the elderly individual.

Physical environment

The physical environment may have an impact on an individual's ability to recover from a push or some other perturbation. The physical environment includes:

- the visual surround
- the ground or floor
- the contact between the ground and a person's shoe
- illumination of the environment
- people walking nearby in the environment.

The visual surround refers to the visual characteristics or appearance of the environment as it is seen by *the person*. Characteristics of the visual surround include:

- the size of objects in the area
- the contrast between objects within the environment
- any glare that is present as a result of lighting or reflection
- the colour attributes of objects
- the movement of objects or people
- any other visual input that is perceived by a person's visual system.

Research has evaluated the reactions of people with visual difficulties. An individual with low vision as a result of macular degeneration (a vision disorder impairing the central region of the visual field) exhibits more adaptations when walking over an object having the same colour as the background than when walking over an object whose colour contrasts highly with the background.[30] For an individual with poor peripheral vision, the ability to see movement in the surrounding area (including the sides, top and bottom of the field of vision) will be impaired. Visual difficulties in the periphery will impact on activities such as walking in a shopping area where other people are moving, because without good peripheral vision a person cannot see movement. This problem can be enough to cause a person to be unsteady on his or her feet. Therefore, well planned visual attributes of the environment to improve visual cues, and an understanding of how vision and visual difficulties affect balance, can play an important part in helping a person maintain balance.

The ground may be slippery, shiny, textured, flat or uneven. 'Slipping during various kinds of movement often leads to potentially dangerous incidents of falling.'[31] The ground characteristics impact on the person's ability to see the ground clearly. For example, if two different heights (as would be found on stairs) show no visual or physical differences at the edge, a person with compromised vision might have difficulty seeing the difference in height. Lack of any contrast on stairs could lead to a fall due to the person's inability to see the depth or the difference in height between the surfaces.

When surfaces such as smooth, wet floors are in contact with a person's shoe, a slip may result. Research conducted to evaluate the friction characteristics between the floor and a shoe, indicates that both static and dynamic friction are important for balance control. Static friction is friction between two surfaces when no movement is occurring between the surfaces. Dynamic friction occurs when there is movement between two surfaces.

Friction is dependent on two characteristics. The first characteristic is the force exerted by an object downwards on the contact surface. This force acts opposite to the direction of motion. If a box is sitting on a surface and is pushed, but no movement occurs, then the static friction is greater than the exerted force. If movement occurs, then there is dynamic friction. Dynamic friction is a friction force which works against the motion.[32] The maximum static friction is greater than dynamic friction. Once something, or someone, starts to slip there will be less friction to hold them in place.

The second feature of friction is the characteristics of the surfaces involved. There are always two surfaces pushing against one another, for example, a shoe bottom and the ground, or a cooking pot and a counter surface. The smoother or more slippery the surfaces in contact with each other are, the lower the coefficient of friction between them. It the coefficient is low, there is a chance that there will be movement. Using our examples, the foot could slide on the ground, or someone could slide the cooking pot along the counter surface. If the ground characteristics are rough and the person's shoes are not slippery, the possibility of slipping and falling is decreased. If the pot is sitting on non-slip material rather than on the counter, it will be difficult to move. Thus, the smoothness or roughness of the surfaces coming into contact with one another are important in determining if sliding will occur.

However, there can be a problem as a result of too much, as well as too little friction. If the friction is too great, the person can be stopped by friction between the ground and the foot. This difficulty can occur when someone walks on a soft rug wearing rough-soled shoes. If the person shuffles, the foot may be stopped during walking because of its contact with the floor. The person may be surprised and may fall when the foot does not swing through but stops during walking.

When a person is walking, there is usually some braking force exerted at the point of contact between the foot and the floor as the person puts the foot down after taking a step. At this point, if this force is influenced by too much friction, the person will fall forward, because the foot sticks to the floor. The opposite occurs when the ground is shiny or slippery and the shoe has little tread, causing a low friction coefficient which then allows the shoe to slip along the ground.

The person

Both the abilities and the limitations of an individual affect balance maintenance. Intact sensory and motor systems will probably ensure balance can be maintained under most conditions. However, many of the individuals with whom occupational therapists work do not have normal muscle strength or control, or they lack sensory control. Some people also have a fear of losing balance and falling.[33]

Someone who has experienced or sustained a CVA or stroke can have difficulties that affect stability: loss of muscle control in the lower extremity, and lack of limb stabilisation on the paretic side of the body can cause problems.[34] People who have experienced CVAs can also experience a change in postural sway, standing symmetry and postural activity preceding movements.[35] There can be lower postural performance in individuals with right brain damage than in those whose damage has occurred in the left hemisphere of the brain. There is a hemispheric dominance for spatial attention and/or representation impacting balance.[36]

Researchers who investigated the sitting stability of individuals following spinal cord injury found the individuals lost stability under dynamic conditions even though they were stable in static situations. These results imply that external lateral supports may be needed to improve a person's sitting balance in dynamic situations.[37]

Researchers who have conducted work with individuals who have experienced mild traumatic brain injury implied an association between balance and the cognitive performance, but not between balance and emotional wellbeing. Geurts et al[38] determined that there is an organic, rather than a functional, cause of postural instability following concussion.

Despite the many different physical difficulties affecting a person's balance, stability and safety, it is important to remember a person usually uses available sensory inputs to control and maintain balance. The individual can then perform functional tasks. The therapist can point out the abilities a person has, make suggestions about changing the environment or the footwear, and let the person know what environments may pose a problem to balance.

Occupational demands

The occupations a person performs make many demands on the individual. Motions of the legs and trunk vary with each task and include reaching, stepping and twisting, to name but a few. Postural adjustments are scaled to the expected size of a perturbation. Many people have lifted something that appears to be heavy and have had to make adjustments because the object was actually much lighter than was expected. People also stiffen under highly threatening conditions for maintaining stance, as was demonstrated when people were asked to stand on the edge of an 81 cm high surface compared to standing on a normal ground surface.[39] Figure 6.2 illustrates how people must sometimes walk over obstacles in their paths. Avoiding obstacles successfully requires good balance and motor control, because both feet must successfully clear the object, otherwise a trip or fall could occur. Can you think of ways to help people avoid tripping or falling?

Some researchers suggest movement can be changed to help control balance problems. Other researchers suggest functional reach does not measure dynamic balance. Healthy elderly people, and individuals who were balance impaired as a result of vestibular dysfunction, can have the same functional reach as one another. Evaluation of posture, however, should be interpreted with caution. Many occupations required twisting tasks which can be performed in awkward, asymmetric postures, implying results from upright twisting studies might underestimate the risk of these activities.[40]

Figure 6.2   Obstacle avoidance.

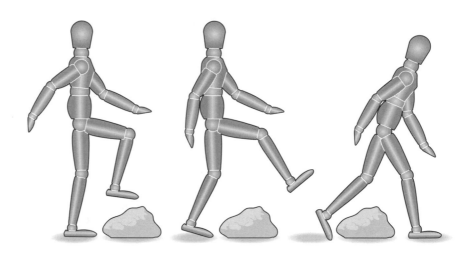

ASSESSING THE POTENTIAL FOR TRIPS AND FALLS

One of the most important things to be able to determine as a therapist, but also one of the most difficult assessments, is evaluating if a person might trip or fall in the future. There are both clinical assessments and research assessments which can be done to determine if a person may fall, although the therapist cannot always be absolutely sure or predict with accuracy whether a trip or fall can occur.

Clinical assessment

Familiarity with balance instruments can be useful when selecting an appropriate clinical tool to institute appropriate prevention programmes such as environmental modifications, or lifestyle modifications.[41] It is appropriate to measure both voluntary and involuntary movement[18] and correlate the results of balance measures with functional mobility and sensory organisation.[17]

Time is frequently used as a measure of a person's ability to maintain balance. When time is used as an objective measure, it does not necessarily offer an assessment of function.[9] Tests of balance should include the ability to maintain a given posture and to ensure stability when the position is changed. The scale should also be applicable for the majority of people, even those with poor postural performance, and should contain items with increasing increments of difficulty.[36] Balance scales should include the assessment of the ability to maintain static and dynamic balance, to control appropriate postures under perturbing conditions, to produce normal movement characteristics, and to adapt balance during perturbations introduced while the subjects are walking.[42] It appears that some physical fitness evaluations provide results that may not be entirely accurate in an individual who has a visual impairment.[43]

Measuring functional reach does not necessarily measure stability and balance. In one research study healthy elderly people and individuals who were balance impaired attained the same functional reach distance.[44] Some results show both motor control patterns and dynamic balance indices correlated well to the extent of mobility impairment, evaluated using the traditional Functional Independence Measure (FIM).[45] Some balance tests are done under extreme conditions that are very challenging, particularly when the therapist is working in ergonomics.[46]

Biomechanical methods have been used to measure balance. For example, the electromyographic patterns of trunk muscles during sitting have been evaluated.[47] Research looking at sit-to-stand in people with hemiplegia and those without a neurological problem, and related data from force plates, including ground reaction forces and centre of pressure data, found that FIM scores correlated with these biomechanical balance indices.[15] Accelerometers measure acceleration. They can be inexpensive, can also be used for balance testing, training and relearning by providing feedback concerning a person's acceleration.

Biomechanical measures can contribute not only to assessment but also to an understanding of the mechanisms of balance control, and to the understanding of ways to treat balance problems and hopefully decrease the number of falls a person has. This is extremely important for individuals who have balance difficulties. The occupational therapist can encourage an individual to return to activities requiring movement to constantly perturb and challenge the balance system.

Potential responses to perturbations

The first type of postural response is anticipatory preparation which occurs when the person expects that there will be a change and a need for balance adjustments. This type of preparation occurs before the perturbation is exerted on the person. Anticipatory control requires fast and fluent execution of movement.[5] Do and colleagues[48] found the control of short swing phase duration in gait resulted in earlier onset latency of stepping to recovery. However, it is also possible that neither step length nor step velocity could induce an earlier onset of stepping. Balance control can include head and trunk coordination.[49] Visual information helps stabilise posture by reducing the variability of the head's position in space for all but the slowest translation frequencies.[50] Gilles et al[51] concluded that prior information does not speed postural responses that differ quantitatively and according to the direction of perturbation balance. Often, there is no opportunity to prepare a response to a potential perturbation. The perturbation occurs and the individual must respond to it after its occurrence. This requires feedforward control, then readjustment. Feedforward control implies information is given to the system. In this case, the feedforward is provided to the individual by the sensory organs and is responded to by the person after the information has been provided.

Strategies can be sought for restoring balance and stability even when slipping occurs unexpectedly.[31] Slipping during walking, however, cannot always be significantly compensated for on the first step after a slip occurs.[24] Trunk inputs from the muscles can be valuable in maintaining balance.[28]

In older individuals there are longer onset times, smaller magnitudes and longer durations of compensation, compared with younger individuals.[17] Individuals with Parkinson's disease had difficulty regaining body equilibrium after unexpected perturbations.[52] They have specific difficulty with leaning back and maintaining balance.[52]

HOW CAN THERAPISTS PREVENT TRIPS AND FALLS OR ALLEVIATE THEIR EFFECTS?

In order to help prevent a trip or fall, change must occur in whichever factor is causing the problem: the environment, the person, or the occupation. The possibility of a fall can be reduced by modifying these factors that affect balance. For example, light can be added to the environment to increase the sensory input to the visual system. In the sit-to-stand situation, one can provide arm rests, a raised seat height, and/or use mechanical elevation devices. Regardless of the seat height or use of the mechanical elevating devices, chairs should have arm rests.[53]

Rehabilitation or training can help individuals for whom balance could potentially become a problem. Early intervention is important to maintain the individual's physical activity and prevent the cycle of inactivity, increased dysfunction, and dependence occurring when there is a loss of confidence in walking.[54] The activities should be context-specific postural responses that can be either relearned or retrained following a stroke or other problems that affect balance. Unfortunately, deficits in the sequences and timing of stabilising muscular responses can be resistant to adaptation. If the individual is aware of an ensuing balance disturbance, the initiation of responses occurs with voluntary motion.[34]

Vision and proprioception are both considered to be important in this area. Visual information is important in maintaining a fixed position of the head and trunk in space as well as for understanding the relationship of the person to the environment. Appropriate information can be sufficient to produce appropriate patterns between the support surfaces and the legs.[50]

Physical and sports activities provide important positive assistance for postural control and appear to be useful for elderly individuals even if activity has not been a lifelong habit.[26] Regular walking can also be incorporated into strategies for improving balance in the elderly.[21] Proprioception exercises appear to have a positive impact on balance control.[55] Rehabilitation appears to improve sitting balance in individuals with spinal cord injuries.[56] Touching an object in the environment with the hand appears to assist in the regulation of normal posture as well as assisting in inherently unstable postures.[57] Thus, for individuals with balance problems a number of solutions in training, with a variety of methods appear to be useful. Occupational therapists should consider incorporating these activities into a balance training programme.

There is little information available in the research to suggest changes in the person's occupation that can produce fewer occurrences of trips and falls. It appears, though, that contact of the hand with a stationary surface can be a way to control postural sway in normal individuals, even when the force is inadequate to change the amount of body motion. Research has found that during quiet stance, light touch of the finger on a stationary surface can be more effective than vestibular function for minimising sway in posture.[58] When engaging in occupations, one must take into account the physical environment, the types of movements required by the individual, and the velocity with which those movements must be made. The occupation can be adapted to encourage postural control by providing a solid surface that a person can hold onto to balance. By ensuring the ground characteristics are not slippery, uneven or too rough, safe balancing can be encouraged.

SUMMARY

When promoting safe balance, it is important to incorporate the physical environment, the person and the occupation in which the person is engaged. This area of research and clinical practice is important because of the large number of falls occurring annually and the devastating effect these falls have. The clinical occupational therapist evaluates the movements, the environment and the occupation on which the person is working, to ensure the lowest potential for trips or falls to occur.

QUESTIONS BASED ON THE CASE

Consider yourself to be in the occupational therapy student's position. Answer the following questions, using the information from this chapter and other reading you have found useful.

1. Prioritise the physical problems Ms Henderson has because of her traumatic brain injury. Order them according to what you think are the priorities. Now, think again. This time, consider them in relation to Ms Henderson's thinking. Are the priorities that you have as a professional any different from those that Ms Henderson would have?
2. How have her physical problems, particularly her balance, impacted on her occupations?
3. What are the safety issues for Ms Henderson?
4. How would you address Ms Henderson's priorities?
5. How might you recommend Ms Henderson change her physical environment?
6. What further information would you need to help Ms Henderson and how would you get this vital information?
7. What adaptive devices would you recommend to Ms Henderson for her to improve her balance?
8. Do you think Ms Henderson will eventually return to her apartment and be safe there?

Laboratory Exercises

1. Balance is influenced by feedback and sensory information. To mimic sensory losses, do the following activities. Maintain static balance while you are doing them. Be sure you have someone standing close to you in case you lose your balance. Do the following:
   a. Take your shoes off and stand on a solid surface.
   b. Find a very soft, thick cushion. A wheelchair cushion made of temprafoam, or an equivalent cushion, is useful for this activity. Stand on the cushion.

continued overpage

c. Stand on the cushion with your eyes closed.

d. Stand on the cushion with your eyes closed and your head back, with your face towards the ceiling.

Answer the following questions about the balance activities you just did:

(i) Which of the activities caused you the most difficulty?

(ii) Can you think of physical problems that might impede balance in the same ways you just experienced?

2. You will learn the concept of stability margins from this exercise. There should be people standing in front of and behind you, so you do not fall if you lose your balance. Do the following activities. Let the person pushing you decide what order to do them and do not let that person tell you ahead of time how hard he or she is going to push.

a. Have the person behind you push very gently against your back. Have people observe what your physical response to the activity is.

b. The person should push you a bit harder.

c. You could be pushed to the point at which you must take a step to maintain your balance.

3. Relate your responses to the above exercise in which you were pushed (had your balance perturbed) to the information in this chapter. Is there a similarity between your responses and those responses reported in the research? What could be the implications of a person with instability, such as Ms Henderson, experiences, being pushed to their stability limits?

4. Balance can be either static or dynamic. For a dynamic balance exercise, try walking with your eyes closed and your head tilted back. How do you maintain your balance? Can you maintain your balance at all?

5. Examine the surfaces of the bottom of three pairs of shoes. Are they slippery or do they have treads on them? Both types of soles can cause problems. Why?

6. If you live in a cold climate, you will probably have experienced walking outside in icy or snowy conditions. Do you know what your balance corrections are for these conditions? What sort of adaptations do you use to be sure you do not fall?

7. Think of someone working in a kitchen:

a. What would be the balance difficulty for people reaching above their head?

b. What happens if someone has to reach far in front of them for objects?

c. What happens if the objects are easily within reach?

d. Knowing the differences between these activities, how would you help someone with balance difficulties organise a workspace to reduce the chances of falling?

8. Falls happen in individuals who are older:

a. What objects would you examine in the home of an individual who has balance difficulties?

b. What adaptations would you make to a home to help reduce falls?

c. How would you suggest the person change their performance of activities of daily living?

REFERENCES

1. Woollacott MH, Shumway-Cook A. Changes in posture control across the life span – a systems approach. Phys Ther 1990; 70(12):799–807.
2. Kavounoudias A, Gilhodes JC, Roll R, Roll JP. From balance regulation to body orientation: two goals for muscle proprioceptive information processing? Exp Brain Res 1999; 124(1):80–88.
3. Horak FB, Henry SM, Shumway-Cook A. Postural perturbations: new insights for treatment of balance disorders. Phys Ther 1997; 77(5):517–533.
4. Szturm T, Fallang B. Effects of varying acceleration of platform translation and toes-up rotations on the pattern and magnitude of balance reactions in humans. J Vestib Res 1998; 8(5):381–397.
5. Toussaint HM, Michies YM, Faber MN, et al. Scaling anticipatory postural adjustments dependent on confidence of load estimation in a bi-manual whole-body lifting task. Exp Brain Res 1998; 120(1):85–94.
6. Abe M, Yamada N. Postural coordination patterns associated with the swinging frequency of arms. Exp Brain Res 2001; 139(1):120–125.
7. Adolph KE, Avolio AM. Walking infants adapt locomotion to changing body dimensions. J Exp Psychol Hum Percept Perform 2000; 26(3):1148–1166.
8. Agostino R, Sanes JN, Hallett M. Motor skill learning in Parkinson's disease. J Neurol Sci 1996; 139(2):218–226.
9. Wagner SG, Pfeifer A, Cranfield TL, Craik RL. The effects of ageing on muscle strength and function: a review of the literature. Physiother Theory Pract 1994; 10(1):9–16.
10. Laporte DM, Chan D, Sveistrup H. Rising from sitting in elderly people, part 1: implications of biomechanics and physiology. Br J Occup Ther 1999; 62(1):36–42.
11. Alexander NB, Grunawalt JC, Carlos S, Augustine J. Bed mobility task performance in older adults. J Rehabil Res Dev 2000; 37(5):633–638.
12. Black K, Zafonte R, Millis S, et al. Sitting balance following brain injury: does it predict outcome? Brain Inj 2000; 14(2):141–152.
13. Brown LA, Shumway-Cook A, Woollacott MH. Attentional demands and postural recovery: the effects of aging. J Gerontol Biol Sci Med Sci 1999; 54(4): M165–M171.
14. Izquierdo M, Aguado X, Gonzalez R, et al. Maximal and explosive force production capacity and balance performance in men of different ages. Eur J Appl Physiol Occup Physiol 1999; 79(3):260–267.
15. Angulo-Kinzler RM, Mynark RG, Koceja DM. Soleus H-reflex gain in elderly and young adults: modulation due to body position. J Gerontol Biol Sci Med Sci 1998; 53(2):M120–M125.
16. Brauer SG, Burns YR, Galley P. A prospective study of laboratory and clinical measures of postural stability to predict community-dwelling fallers. J Gerontol Biol Sci Med Sci 2000; 55(8):M469–M476.
17. Tang PF, Woollacott MH. Inefficient postural responses to unexpected slips during walking in older adults. J Gerontol Biol Sci Med Sci 1998; 53(6):M471–M480.
18. Luchies CW, Wallace D, Pazdur R, et al. Effects of age on balance assessment using voluntary and involuntary step tasks. J Gerontol Biol Sci Med Sci 1999; 54A(3): M140–M144.
19. Simoneau M, Teasdale N, Bourdin C, et al. Aging and postural control: postural perturbations caused by changing the visual anchor. J Am Geriatr Soc 1999; 47(2): 235–240.
20. Andersson G, Yardley L, Luxon L. A dual-task study of interference between mental activity and control of balance. Am J Otol 1998; 19(5):632–637.
21. Brooke-Wavell K, Athersmith LE, Jones PR, Masud T. Brisk walking and postural stability: a cross-sectional study in postmenopausal women. Gerontology 1998; 44(5): 288–292.
22. Bulbulian R, Hargan ML. The effect of activity history and current activity on static and dynamic postural balance in older adults. Physiol Behav 2000; 70(3–4):319–325.
23. Brooke-Wavell K, Perrett LK, Howarth PA, Haslam RA. Influence of the visual environment on the postural stability in healthy older women. Gerontology 2002; 48(5):293–297.

24. Tang PF, Moore S, Woollacott MH. Correlation between two clinical balance measures in older adults: functional mobility and sensory organization test. J Gerontol Biol Sci Med Sci 1998; 53(2):M140–M146.

25. Archambault P, Pigeon P, Feldman AG, Levin MF. Recruitment and sequencing of different degrees of freedom during pointing movements involving the trunk in healthy and hemiparetic subjects. Exp Brain Res 1999; 126(1):55–67.

26. Perrin PP, Gauchard GC, Perrot C, Jeandel C. Effects of physical and sporting activities on balance control in elderly people. Br J Sports Med 1999; 33(2):121–126.

27. Robinovitch SN, Cronin T. Perception of postural limits in elderly nursing home and day care participants. J Gerontol Biol Sci Med Sci 1999; 54A(3):B124–B131.

28. Allum JH, Honegger F. Interactions between vestibular and proprioceptive inputs triggering and modulating human balance-correcting responses differ across muscles. Exp Brain Res 1998; 121(4):478–494.

29. Burtner PA, Woollacott MH, Qualls C. Stance balance control with orthoses in a group of children with spastic cerebral palsy. Dev Med Child Neurol 1999; 41(11):748–757.

30. Spaulding SJ, Patla AE, Rietdyk S, et al. Gait adaptations during dark and light adaptation in individuals with age-related maculopathy. Gait Posture 1995; 3(4):227–235.

31. Pai YC, Iqbal K. Simulated movement termination for balance recovery: can movement strategies be sought to maintain stability in the presence of slipping or forced sliding? J Biomech 1999; 32(8):779–786.

32. Hall SJ. Basic biomechanics. 1st edn. Toronto: Mosby Year Book; 1991.

33. Yardley L. Fear of imbalance and falling. Rev Clin Gerontol 1998; 8(1):23–29.

34. Di Fabio RP. Adaptation of postural stability following stroke. Top Stroke Rehabil 1997; 3(4):62–75.

35. Leonard E. Balance tests and balance responses: performance changes following a CVA. A review of the literature. Physiother Can 1990; 42(2):68–72.

36. Benaim C, Perennou DA, Villy J, et al. Validation of a standardized assessment of postural control in stroke patients: the Postural Assessment Scale for Stroke Patients (PASS). Stroke 1999; 30(9):1862–1868.

37. Kamper DG, Barin K, Parnianpour M, et al. Preliminary investigation of the lateral postural stability of spinal cord-injured individuals subjected to dynamic perturbations. Spinal Cord 1999; 37(1):40–46.

38. Geurts AC, Knoop JA, van Limbeek J. Is postural control associated with mental functioning in the persistent postconcussion syndrome? Arch Phys Med Rehabil 1999; 80(2):144–149.

39. Carpenter MG, Frank JS, Silcher CP, Peysar GW. The influence of postural threat on the control of upright stance. Exp Brain Res 2001; 138(2):210–218.

40. Marras WS, Davis KG, Granata KP. Trunk muscle activities during asymmetric twisting motions. J Electromyogr Kinesiol 1998; 8(4):247–256.

41. Whitney SL, Poole JL, Cass SP. A review of balance instruments for older adults. Am J Occup Ther 1998; 52(8):666–671.

42. Patla A, Frank J, Winter D. Assessment of balance control in the elderly: major issues. Physiother Can 1990; 42(2):89–97.

43. Skaggs S, Hopper C. Individuals with visual impairments: a review of psychomotor behavior. Adapt Phys Activity Q 1996; 13(1):16–26.

44. Wernick-Robinson M, Krebs DE, Giorgetti MM. Functional reach: does it really measure dynamic balance? Arch Phys Med Rehabil 1999; 80(3):262–269.

45. Lee MY, Wong MK, Tang FT, et al. New quantitative and qualitative measures on functional mobility prediction for stroke patients. J Med Eng Technol 1998; 22(1):14–24.

46. Holbein MA, Chaffin DB. Stability limits in extreme postures: effects of load positioning, foot placement, and strength. Hum Factors 1997; 39(3):456–468.

47. Zedka M, Kumar S, Narayan Y. Electromyographic response of the trunk muscles to postural perturbation in sitting subjects. J Electromyogr Kinesiol 1998; 8(1):3–10.

48. Do MC, Schneider C, Chong RK. Factors influencing the quick onset of stepping following postural perturbation. J Biomech 1999; 32(8):795–802.

49. Nicholas SC, Doxey-Gasway DD, Paloski WH. Investigator: Paloski WH. A link-segment model of upright human posture for analysis of head–trunk coordination. J Vestib Res 1998; 8(3):187–200.

50. Buchanan JJ, Horak FB. Investigator: Peterson BW. Emergence of postural patterns as a function of vision and translation frequency. J Neurophysiol 1999; 81(5):2325–2339.
51. Gilles M, Wing AM, Kirker SG. Lateral balance organisation in human stance in response to a random or predictable perturbation. Exp Brain Res 1999; 124(2):137–144.
52. Immisch I, Bandmann O, Quintern J, Straube A. Different postural reaction patterns for expected and unexpected perturbations in patients with idiopathic Parkinson's disease and other parkinsonian syndromes. Eur J Neurol 1999; 6(5):549–554.
53. Munro BJ, Steele JR. Facilitating the sit-to-stand transfer: a review. Phys Ther Rev 1998; 3(4):213–224.
54. Vandervoort A, Hill K, Sandrin M, Vyse VM. Mobility impairment and falling in the elderly. Physiother Can 1990; 42(2):99–107.
55. Gauchard GC, Jeandel C, Tessier A, Perrin PP. Beneficial effect of proprioceptive physical activities on balance control in elderly human subjects. Neurosci Lett 1999; 273(2):81–84.
56. Seelen HA, Potten YJ, Adam JJ, et al. Postural motor programming in paraplegic patients during rehabilitation. Ergonomics 1998; 41(3):302–316.
57. Clapp S, Wing AM. Light touch contribution to balance in normal bipedal stance. Exp Brain Res 1999; 125(4):521–524.
58. Lackner JR, DiZio P, Jeka J, et al. Investigator: Lackner JR. Precision contact of the fingertip reduces postural sway of individuals with bilateral vestibular loss. Exp Brain Res 1999; 126(4):459–466.

Chapter 7

Environmental demands on occupations

CHAPTER CONTENTS

Occupations do not occur in a vacuum. We have to perform occupations in an environment. We know the environment can include our homes, our places of work, buildings of worship or the outside world. The environment becomes a large presence for people who live with physical difficulties. They may not be able to get through doorways when they are using wheelchairs. They may not be able to go to movies with their friends because there is no lift to the theatre or no accessible toilets. They may not be able to visit their families because they cannot get on trains.

Occupational therapists must consider the environment in which occupations occur. They must be able to evaluate the environment for an individual and suggest alterations to make occupations possible. The purpose of this chapter is to discuss environments and what we can do to make them work to enhance rather than hinder people's engagement in occupations.

While you are studying the information about environments, consider the contents of the following case. There will be questions at the end of the chapter, based on integrating the material in the case with information about environments, adaptations and universal design.

CASE STUDY: PHILIP SMITH

Philip Smith is a 17-year-old boy who is attending secondary school and is participating in a normal classroom environment with peers his own age. Philip is working on fewer subjects in school than his friends are. He has cerebral palsy with spasticity which slows down his ability to complete projects, but he has no difficulty learning, given enough time and the right environment.

The setting

Philip lives with his mother and his two younger sisters. He visits his father during the weekends. The setting of concern is the environment of Philip's family home. The school is not a problem, because it is wheelchair accessible and it is easy for Philip to get around.

The occupational therapist

The occupational therapist, Maureen O'Brian, works at the regional children's centre and has been working with the adolescent population for 15 years. She is primarily involved with augmentative communication, mobility and issues related to the environment. Most of her work is done in the homes of the people she works with. She works with other therapists whose focus is the school setting.

The individual

Philip is a teenager with the typical issues that teenagers have. He struggles for autonomy from his mother. He usually gets along with his siblings, but they have typical sibling fights. When Philip was younger his mother spent time dealing with the emotional issues that sometimes come with beginning to raise a child with physical difficulties, but she is fine with it now and interacts with Philip in much the same way as with her other children.

Physical abilities

Philip's cerebral palsy has affected all of his body, so he has limited use of his arms and legs and he cannot speak. He has no other physical problems and because he and his mother have managed the cerebral palsy well, he has had few hospitalisations as a result of related problems, and he has had no skin breakdowns.

Philip uses augmentative communication to communicate with his friends, surf on the internet and do his homework. He has relatively good use of his hands and his manual dexterity is functional enough that he can use a normal keyboard on a computer.

Philip is extremely limited in his physical functioning. He has, as mentioned previously, enough use of his upper extremities to let him use an augmentative communication system with a computer as designed by the occupational therapist. He does use a wheelchair, but until recently has been using a manual model and has had to be pushed by someone else, because he could not propel it himself. He has been given funding by a private agency to help his mother purchase a powered wheelchair that he and the occupational therapist expect he will be able to manage independently with a commercial joystick control.

Philip uses many pieces of adaptive equipment throughout his home. He has undergone a number of surgeries to reduce the effect of the spasticity in his legs to help him with his functioning, however, the surgery was not carried out with the expectation that he would be able to walk, but to release contractures and allow for easier care.

Emotional status

Philip has the typical emotional issues of a 17-year-old. He relates to his mother as many adolescents do. He does not seem to have any major emotional issues or problems that are particularly related to his cerebral palsy. He does belong to a group of adolescents with physical disabilites, through the treatment centre, and he enjoys his time with the group members. They have a good time together and all consider one another friends. He also has some friends at school. He does find it frustrating at times though, because his computer access for communication is somewhat slow. It is hard for him to engage his friends in conversation with him because of the slowness. He has made friends through the internet around the world and he enjoys communicating with them.

Philip's mother has been able to teach him good social interaction skills with his methods of communication. He is working his way towards becoming an advocate for people with physical problems.

Exploring issues with Philip

Philip's mother is finding it increasingly difficult to manage him physically, because he has grown to be 6 feet tall and weighs approximately 180 pounds. His spasticity impedes his ability to help his mother when she is doing transfers and helping him with his activities of daily living.

The issues for Philip are the size of his new wheelchair relative to some of the structures in his home. The school environment is not a problem for him. The school that he attends is accessible for him. He has access to a specially designed classroom when he is unable to do activities in his usual classroom, but generally he is involved with his class and uses his augmentative communication system. The larger environment in his city also presents challenges. Even public buildings that are supposed to be wheelchair accessible are not always easy to enter or get around. Public transportation is also a problem, because at his age, Philip does not want to be dependent on his mother to get him from place to place.

Philip and his family have lived in their apartment since he was 7 years old, after his parents divorced. He is very familiar with the building, as are his sisters. The family is extremely reluctant to move at this point. This might have been an option to consider because there may be other more accessible places where he could live. However, the family have been in the apartment for a long time, and they know the manager and the management staff of the apartment building well. There is some willingness on the part of the management to make modifications, if they can be done for a reasonable cost. Philip's mother is not able to afford the changes herself. So the big issue for Philip and his family is to enhance the environment so that he will not be limited when he increases his mobility with his powered wheelchair, or because of his increased size. He has probably not stopped growing yet as he is only 17 years old. There is also the concern that it will become more difficult for him and his mother to manage his physical problems. As the situation remains, there will be a number of issues for him.

The home environment

Philip's home environment is the apartment where he lives with his mother and siblings. The apartment is on the fifteenth floor of a high-rise building in a large urban area. At the moment, Philip is able to manage getting into the building and up to his floor in his wheelchair, using the lift to the apartment. The doors in the apartment are wide enough for him when he enters and manoeuvres throughout the apartment. It is not easy to get around, but the layout of the apartment has been working for him up to this point. However, when he starts to use an adult-size battery-powered wheelchair, there will be many aspects of the apartment that will no longer work for him, because the new wheelchair is much larger. For example, the doorways within the apartment will be barely wide enough, and the bathroom doorway will be too narrow, so he will not be able to get in and out of the bathroom in his wheelchair. The kitchen is functional for him and he does help with meals within his limited capabilities. He is not independent in activities of daily living, primarily due to the spasticity in the proximal joints of his upper extremities and the spasticity in his legs. Since his operations, he has become less dependent. He can move his extremities more readily. His mother finds it is easier to bathe him, to assist him to get dressed, and complete toileting activities with him.

FUNDAMENTAL CONCEPTS FOR UNDERSTANDING THE ENVIRONMENT

> ■ *Adaptable or accessible design:* This means adapting an environment for an individual.[1] Researchers[2] consider that the interpretation of accessibility requires the perspective of both the individual and the community.
> ■ *Barrier-free design:* This is design for a specific group of people, for example design of an accessible school for children who use wheelchairs. Barrier-free design and implementation may be applied to existing buildings.[1]
> ■ *Universal design:* Universal design 'recognizes that people have a range of capabilities and designs need to include this range'.[1]

PHYSICAL ENVIRONMENT

The physical environment can enable people who have physical problems or it can actually increase the handicap a person experiences. For example, a curb without an incorporated ramp will be helpful for someone who has low vision and ambulates while using a cane. The curb can be felt by the cane and will make the person aware that a roadway may be close by. The same curb is a barrier for someone who uses a wheelchair and cannot negotiate a curb with the wheelchair. The physical environment can be a problem for people with physical and cognitive problems. For example, researchers[3] found that for individuals performing occupations after strokes, there can be constant difficulties in dealing with the physical world.

Assistive devices can be considered as useful tools to help individuals perform occupations and interact with the environment,[4] yet these devices can also be considered to cause problems for individuals when they lead other people to view the person differently. Research shows that the presence of physical barriers hampers people with disabilities and increases their handicaps.[5–10] It is important that any analysis of accessibility should consider both the individual and the environment.[11–13]

Accessibility also needs to be considered from a broader perspective.[14] Simply meeting the guidelines for adaptation will not always meet the occupational needs of individuals.[15] Ensuring that environments are functional for people is very important to their wellbeing and ability to participate in occupations.[16] The use of universal design principles is valuable when evaluating and adapting the environment for individuals. Figure 7.1 illustrates this. The possibility of slipping on steps that have very little contrast between them is increased because of the wet, melting snow. Who would find these steps difficult to use? What would you recommend to make them safer? By entering the public arena and working with

Figure 7.1   Steps in winter.
A difficult environment.

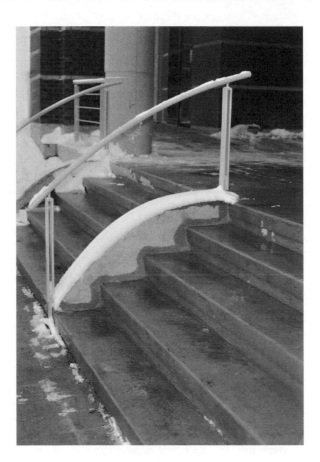

architects, builders and ultimately policy-makers to change the environments, occupational therapists can help establish building standards to meet the needs of people with physical problems, by bearing in mind the concepts of universal design.

When an occupational therapist works with someone who has issues with the environment, it is assumed that the therapist understands some of the constraints that may be inherent in the disability. It can also be important for the therapist to understand some of the mechanical characteristics of the environment and ultimately the sociocultural environment. This understanding of the larger institutional environment and its legal requirements is important and will be touched on briefly here, but further detail is beyond the scope of this book. Readers should check the building specifications of their local government agencies and the legislation that has been passed in their area.

PERSPECTIVES OF THE PERSON USING THE ENVIRONMENT

An environment that enables one person may impede or reduce occupational performance for another. For example, a ramp works as a facilitator for someone who drives a powered mobility device such as a scooter. The same ramp is more difficult to use than stairs for someone who uses crutches for mobility. The ramp becomes a barrier for the person who uses crutches.

Although buildings may be accessible by ramp, this does not always assure the accessibility is ideal. One group of researchers[17] studied the ease of accessibility for wheelchair users of a large urban university. The researchers found that the distances travelled between lecture theatres by students who used wheelchairs were longer than those travelled by ambulatory students. The time the students took to travel between lectures was an average of 17 minutes. This was almost twice as long as the time taken by ambulatory students. For those wheelchair users, it was not possible to reach lectures in a timely fashion. The authors suggested that 'certain administrative changes might assist in improving the ease of accessibility. Architectural adaptations, although more costly, might also prove to be effective.'

Meeting criteria outlined by a country's building standards does not always ensure equal access to the environment. The therapist must examine the accessibility of the environment from the perspective of ease of use, safety, quality, and whether or not it decreases effort and time for mobility for the individual.

ASSESSMENT

The therapist's decision to assess aspects of the environment can be determined by the environments and occupations that are required by the individual. Assessment of architectural elements as sources of stress has been carried out extensively in the workplace in terms of biomechanical parameters such as desk height. The evaluation of architectural components has also been applied in the home settings of people with disabilities.[18]

Occupational therapists evaluating environments must remember that people not only ambulate or use wheelchairs in these settings, they also perform occupations. Occupations are rarely static, but require movement, involve multi-dimensional tasks, and include doing activities over time; so to assess the environment without taking into account a person's occupations within that space may reduce the meaningfulness or usefulness of the assessment. As Rigby and Letts have expressed it:[19] 'The relationship between people and their environments are considered to be dynamic (ever-changing in both directions), complex and inter-dependent'; and 'Evaluation formats range from simple to complex, depending on the therapists' and patients' needs.'[19]

BUILDING STANDARDS

Standards associations in many countries establish minimum acceptable criteria for buildings for people who need specific requirements. In the United States, the *Accessibility Guidelines for Buildings and Facilities* is published by the American National Standards Institute (available at http://www.access-board.gov/adaag/html/adaag.htm)[20] This document notes standards to make buildings more easily usable by people with disabilities.

The World Health Organisation established a nomenclature and checklist; the *International Classification of Functioning, Disability, and Health*.[21] The United Nations has created a manual: *Accessibility for the Disabled. A Design Manual for a Barrier Free Environment*.[22]

Environmental barriers can be present, even when rules are followed, because people's occupations vary, as do their body shapes and sizes. Actual functional accessibility is made evident by a person who uses a wheelchair trying to access a building and perform the occupations that they need or want to do in that space.

PRINCIPLES OF UNIVERSAL DESIGN

Much of the practice of redesigning the environment, as it is conducted by the occupational therapist, involves helping individuals enhance their environments to facilitate occupations. Universal design is a broader concept implying that a particular structure or space can be used by people with many different needs. Universal design, by definition, is design created not for the average person, but for people with a wide range of abilities. Universal design can be applied to a variety of public environments, such as office buildings, theatres, parks, urban planning and websites.[1]

There are a number of attributes of universal design.[23] These can be summed up in the seven principles of universal design as outlined by North Carolina State University in 1997.[24] Universal design incorporates design principles that provide:

- equitable use, such that the design can be used and marketed to people of diverse abilities
- flexibility, so it can be useful for individual preferences and abilities
- simplicity and intuitiveness, so it is easy to understand regardless of the user's current abilities
- perceptible information, so the design communicates necessary information for the user
- error tolerance, so adverse events and hazards are minimised
- low physical effort, so that the design can be used comfortably and efficiently
- size and space for approach and use, so that there is no difficulty with using the space due to limitations of its size and regardless of the user's body size, posture or mobility.

Universal design concepts are used in planning new environments rather than in adapting pre-existing structures. One project, the barrier-free suburb of Marjala in Finland, has been designed for a multitude of individuals. The designers took the lifespan for many people with a variety of needs into consideration.[25] This community was designed by professionals together with citizens and is considered an excellent example of implemented universal design.

Traditionally, occupational therapists have not been involved consistently in the design of these public facilities, although there are exceptions in some communities. But with their understanding of the occupational requirements of people and their increasing comprehension of movement parameters and biomechanics, occupational therapists could, conceivably, make a valuable contribution to the planning and creation of environments using universal design. The creators of universal design spaces, in their goal to have their designs reflect the needs of users, benefit from input from these consumers and from occupational therapists, who work closely with users and frequently work from an individual-centred perspective.

HOME ENVIRONMENTS

When environmental characteristics do not match the physical capacities of an individual, independence may not be possible. Working on changes to an individual's environments, as well as contributing to universal design issues, can both be fields of activity for occupational therapists.

Environmental changes can benefit not only people with physical difficulties, but also their caregivers. Researchers[23] have found a negative correlation between back disability in mothers and dependence level of children with muscular dystrophies. The work of these researchers suggests back health programmes and arrangements to make the home more accessible for children with disabilities, should be added to neuromuscular rehabilitation programmes. Unfortunately, some research on students with difficulties focuses on the students' needs, and fails to consider the environment. If the effects of the environment are not taken into account, students may still be restricted in their ability to go where they would like to go and do what is meaningful for them. If adequate environmental adaptations are not provided, children may be excluded or restricted from participation in some activities.[26,27] For example, if a playground is not adapted so a child with low vision can use it, that child will be excluded from exploring and playing as other children do.

Mothers who are wheelchair users do not always have the freedom or resources to seek out living situations or modify space to meet their needs. However, they do use strategies to gain control over their environments, thus enabling autonomy and participation.[27] For example, mothers can have cribs rebuilt to open from the side so they can reach their infants, and table legs can be shortened or tabletops raised for ease of use.

COMMUNITY ENVIRONMENTS

Environmental settings can impede or enhance mobility for children as well as adults. Palisano et al[28] found that children with cerebral palsy were less dependent on mobility at home compared to in the school setting. In contrast, they were more dependent when outdoors or in the community. This research can trigger our thinking to consider all aspects of occupations. Occupational therapists must keep in mind that different environments

Figure 7.2 A challenging environment. The Drakensburg Mountains in South Africa.

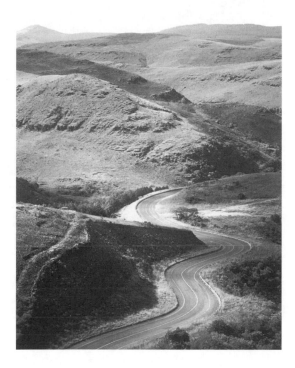

afford different levels of occupational demand. Figure 7.2 shows a rugged environment that would provide quite a challenge for someone with walking difficulties. Think about the environment where you live. Would some people have difficulty getting around in it? What could be done to make it easier for them?

SUMMARY

Occupational therapists should have an understanding of the environment. They must evaluate environmental demands and make recommendations to enhance a person's occupational functioning. Beyond that, it is increasingly clear that therapists need to become more aware of the input they can provide to architects and builders. Lastly, therapists should make a positive impact on design. They need to be involved in groups framing recommendations and legislation to bring in the concepts of universal designs.

Researchers[9] suggest that facilitating social participation by people who use wheelchairs, should focus on personal assistance, assistive technology, and health promotion and fitness, as well as on the built environment.

When an occupational therapist works with someone who has issues with the environment, it is assumed that the therapist understands some of the constraints that may be inherent in the disability. The therapist needs also to understand aspects of the physical environment and the sociocultural environment.

QUESTIONS BASED ON THE CASE

1. What is the primary issue for Philip? Do you think that Philip's problems can be alleviated by modifying his current apartment environment?
2. For Philip living in a small three bedroom apartment, what do you think will be the main environmental issues? Some of them, including door widths and bathroom accessibility have been mentioned, but there may be others you would want to consider.
3. Find a home assessment that would meet the needs of an individual with Philip's particular problems. See if you can get access to a similar apartment and try the assessment out in that environment.
4. Environmental issues have been discussed. What other issues, such as adaptive equipment, might be useful for Philip?
5. What do you think will make the biggest impact on Philip's quality of life?
6. Do you think Philip and his family will have to move?
7. Philip's mother does not have much money. If Philip's family lived in your community, would funds be available, either from the government or from the private sector, if Philip's mother and the occupational therapist applied for it?

Laboratory Exercise: Examples of Environmental Demands on Occupations

1. Each individual needs to have a dwelling and the home is the main environment for many people. Consider your own environment. Ask yourself if it would be possible for a friend who uses a wheelchair to come and visit you in your current living accommodation.
2. If for some reason you were to become physically disabled or were living with someone who became physically disabled, and a wheelchair was required, would your current residence be accessible? If not, would you be able to accommodate in order to function within the environment? If not, what would the alternatives be?
3. When you are doing this exercise, it would be wise to consider all of the equipment required, as well as doorways and other physical features. The home environment is not meant to isolate a person; it should allow the person to perform occupations within it. Ask yourself if you could perform all your current occupations in your living space if you needed to do them while sitting in a wheelchair. The heights of different pieces of furniture may require different methods of functioning. What sort of things would you have difficulty with and what would be some of the solutions that would help you perform your occupations? You should also consider how you could engage in your usual occupations using crutches or a walker.

REFERENCES

1. Ringeart L. Universal design of the built environment to enable occupational performance. In: Letts L, Rigby P, Stewart D, eds. Using environments to enable occupational performance. Thorofare, NJ: Slack; 2003.

2. Jensen G, Iwarsson S, Stahl A. Theoretical understanding and methodological challenges in accessibility assessments, focusing the environmental component: an example from travel chains in urban public bus transport. Disabil Rehabil 2002; 24(5):231–242.

3. Lampinen J, Tham K. Interaction with the physical environment in everyday occupation after stroke: a phenomenological study of persons with visuospatial agnosia. Scand J Occup Ther 2003; 10(4):147–156.

4. McMillen A, Soderberg S. Disabled persons' experience of dependence on assistive devices. Scand J Occup Ther 2002; 9(4):176–183.

5. Chen VT, Baruch LD, Scharf PT, et al. Adaptive housing: remodeling considerations for the disabled. J Burn Care Rehabil 1990; 11(4):352–360.

6. Odette F, Yoshida KK, Israel P, et al. Barriers to wellness activities for Canadian women with physical disabilities. Health Care Women Int 2003; 24(2):125–134.

7. Reid D, Angus J, McKeever P, Miller KL. Home is where their wheels are: experiences of women wheelchair users. Am J Occup Ther 2003; 57(2):186–195.

8. Newman S. The living conditions of elderly Americans. Gerontologist 2003; 43(1): 99–109.

9. Meyers AR, Anderson JJ, Miller DR, et al. Barriers, facilitators, and access for wheelchair users: substantive and methodologic lessons from a pilot study of environmental effects. Soc Sci Med 2002; 55(8):1435–1446.

10. Schopp LH, Sanford TC, Hagglund KJ, et al. Removing service barriers for women with physical disabilities: promoting accessibility in the gynecologic care setting. J Midwifery Womens Health 2002; 47(2):74–79.

11. Iwarsson S, Stahl A. Accessibility, usability and universal design – positioning and definition of concepts describing person–environment relationships. Disabil Rehabil 2003; 25(2):57–66.

12. Picking C, Pain H. Home adaptations: user perspectives on the role of professionals. Br J Occup Ther 2003; 66(1):2–8.

13. Collins F, Smith K. Factors to consider when purchasing a stairlift. Int J Ther Rehabil 2004; 10(9):417– 418.

14. Hawkins R, Stewart S. Changing rooms: the impact of adaptations on the meaning of home for a disabled person and the role of occupational therapists in the process. Br J Occup Ther 2002; 65(2):81–87.

15. Winfield J. Best adaptation redeeming people's homes: enlightened occupational therapy. Br J Occup Ther 2003; 66(8):376–377.

16. Froehlich K, Nary DE, White GW. Identifying barriers to participation in physical activity for women with disabilities. Sci Psychosoc Process 2002; 15(1):21–29.

17. Losinsky LO, Levi T, Saffey K, Jelsma J. An investigation into the physical accessibility to wheelchair bound students of an institution of higher education in South Africa. Disabil Rehabil 2003; 25(7):305–308.

18. Sanford JA, Pynoos J, Tejral A, Browne A. Development of a comprehensive assessment for delivery of home modifications. Phys Occup Ther Geriatr 2002; 20(2):43–55.

19. Rigby P, Letts L. Environment and occupational performance: theoretical considerations. In: Letts L, Rigby P, Stewart D, eds. Using environments to enable occupational performance. Thorofare, NJ: Slack; 2003.

20. American National Standards Institute. Accessibility guidelines for buildings and facilities. ANSI; 2002. Online. Available: http://www.access-board.gov/adaag/html/adaag.htm.

21. World Health Organisation. International classification of function, disability and health. Geneva: WHO; 2001.

22. United Nations. Accessibility for the disabled. A design manual for a barrier free environment. 2003. Online. Available: http://www.un.org/esa/socdev/enable/designm/index.html.

23. Duger T, Yilmaz O, Aki E, et al. The environmental barriers of children with muscular dystrophies and its effect on mother's low back pain. [sic] Disabil Rehabil 2003; 25(20):1187–1192.

24. Story M. Principles of universal design. 1st edn. New York: McGraw-Hill; 2001.
25. Ikonen-Graafmans TSK, Graafmans JAM. The barrier-free suburb of Marjala in Finland: the city for all – the Marjala Model. Technol Disabil 2003; 15(3):201–204.
26. Hemmingson H, Borell L. Environmental barriers in mainstream schools. Child Care Health Dev 2002; 28(1):57–63.
27. Heywood F. Adaptation policies especially for children: key factors for effective outcomes. J Integr Care 2003; 11(1):22–27.
28. Palisano RJ, Tieman BL, Walter SD, et al. Effect of environmental setting on mobility methods of children with cerebral palsy. Dev Med Child Neurol 2003; 45(2):113–120.

Chapter 8

Ergonomics: the study of work occupations

co-authored by

Lynn Shaw

Ergonomics is the study of work occupations. Ergonomics has been defined as the theoretical and fundamental understanding of human behaviour and performance in purposeful systems; and the application of that understanding to the design of interactions in the context of real settings.[1] Therapists working with clients need to consider a number of aspects of work when applying ergonomic principles in the workplace. A broad understanding of factors is needed to determine the interaction of issues that may predispose someone to a work-related injury. Areas for evaluation include: the occupation (e.g. job tasks and performance expectations), the environment (e.g. workplace setting where work is performed, including equipment used and physical considerations); and the person. In Figure 8.1 an older woman is making pots from clay. Doing this work has allowed her to make a living in a place where it is difficult to do so. An occupational therapist with an understanding of biomechanics could help her continue her work by providing suggestions to make it easier for her. Can you think of postures and work positions that would make it easier for someone to sit and work with clay every day? The person needs to have the physical, cognitive and emotional skills to successfully perform work.

These factors and domains need to be examined when interacting with an injured worker.[2] For example, a worker could be recovering from an injury such as carpal tunnel syndrome that was contracted in the work environment. The occupational therapist would need to work with the person, the person's occupations and the environment in order to assist recovery and reduce the chances of repetitive strain injuries occurring again. Another example would be working with someone with a spinal cord injury who requires changes to a work environment. In each case, the therapist considers the interaction of factors about the occupations

Figure 8.1   Making a pot.

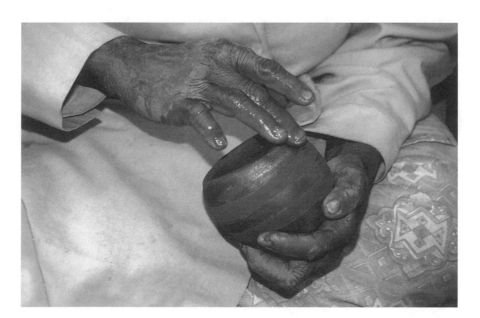

performed, the work environment and the abilities of the person. Only then can adaptations be made enabling the worker to carry out job demands successfully. In other situations, the therapist may be involved with assisting a person with a disability, such as cerebral palsy, to enter the workforce for the first time. All of these aspects of interacting therapeutically with the worker may be part of an occupational therapist's assessment and intervention. Each of them will require slightly different skills from the therapist. At present, there is more research available to therapists to help them understand evaluating the work environment, potential work-related injuries, and processes for returning a worker to the workforce than there is about helping someone with a predisposing difficulty enter the workforce.

Ergonomics has most often been thought of as it relates to heavy industry. Traditionally, research in ergonomics focused on admissible weights for lifting and ways to reduce injuries that may occur in heavy industry. However, within the last couple of decades, the emphasis on technology has led to an increase in worker-related problems occurring due to the predominant use of computers or video display terminals. In effect, research and applications of ergonomic principles have become more widespread. Now, research is expanding into sedentary work environments in which evaluations are needed to understand how to improve the design of workstations for people who use computers, and how to help workers with acquired repetitive strain injuries.

CASE STUDY: MS KATRINA ZELASNIK

Ms Katrina Zelasnik is a 35-year-old woman who is employed by her uncle, Mr Zelasnik. He owns a plate glass retail company. The company owns a house in a residential district not far from the hardware store and other construction companies. The business sells replacement glass for windows, specialty glass for privacy, and many other types of glass. Ms Zelasnik's position is as assistant manager in the store. She has juvenile rheumatoid arthritis and has managed some of the problems associated with that condition since she was 7 years old. Within the past 5 years she has had both knees replaced and may need to consider other joint replacements as the disease progresses. Currently, she fatigues easily and has difficulty with joint inflammation. Subsequently, she has asked for assistance from an occupational therapist to help her adapt her workplace.

The occupational therapist

The occupational therapist is Ms Romana Czainski, who is employed by a private practice occupational therapy company. This private company has five employees, including three occupational therapists and two kinesiologists, each of whom has a minimum of 3 years of experience in the areas of work rehabilitation and ergonomics. For the past 7 years, Ms Czainski has specialised in work-related practice. Her experiences range from working with people who do heavy work at the local oil refineries to working with people who are required to do sedentary occupations such as office or computer work. Much of Ms Czainski's practice involves assisting people who have returned to work after catastrophic injuries. Prior to this job, she gained an understanding of rheumatic disease and treatment through her work with clients in a rheumatology clinic. Based upon her clinical expertise and experiences she was identified as the most suitable member of the company to address Ms Zelasnik's needs.

The client

Ms Zelasnik is an active person, within the constraints of her physical problems. Her family has always encouraged her to do what she can, but also to know her abilities and function within the limits of the disease process. She completed a combined post-secondary education degree in economics and business administration about 10 years ago. Since graduating, she has worked for her uncle. She is an enthusiastic individual and loves spending time with numerous friends who all enjoy her company.

Ms Zelasnik lives in an apartment in close proximity to the business. Presently, her apartment accommodates her physical limitations and functional needs, so she is not concerned with adaptations to her home environment.

Physical abilities

Ms Zelasnik has one health issue – juvenile rheumatoid arthritis. She is very uncomfortable sometimes, especially when her joints are inflamed. When her endurance is low, she tires very easily and experiences more difficulties working. Currently the joint range of motion in her upper extremities is restricted. She can only move her shoulders to about 90° of flexion and abduction. Her elbows are painful when there is inflammation, but she has good range of motion in them at other times. Standing for long periods is also problematic because of pain and stiffness in her hips. Typically, this occurs when she does not get up and move around when she is working. The effects of the disease limit her functioning at work. For example, although she would like to perform well all day, her pain and subsequent decreased mobility interfere with her ability to be consistently productive.

Emotional status and social supports

Ms Zelasnik has come to terms with her disease, although she sometimes finds it frustrating. She does not have any underlying emotional problems; however, at times her reduced mobility hinders her participation socially. At times, she cannot engage in physically demanding activities with her friends such as biking or hiking. However, she belongs to a small peer support group for people with rheumatic diseases. Being involved in this group is helpful because she has met people who have similar difficulties and frustrations. The people in the group consider one another friends. It was through her connection with a member from this group that she learned that an occupational therapist might be helpful in assisting her to adapt her workplace.

Exploring issues with Ms Zelasnik

The predominant, overriding issue for Ms Zelasnik is to see if her workplace and occupations in that environment can be adapted so that she can do her work with less fatigue, pain and frustration. She has told the occupational therapist that although her goal is to make her work environment easier in which to perform her work, she does not want to cause fellow employees inconvenience or create problems through changes made to the workstation set-up. She would also like the occupational therapist to help her find ways to perform tasks more efficiently, considering her limitations and changes in health status.

Evaluating the setting

The therapist conducted a worksite visit to review the environment and to meet Ms Zelasnik and her employer. While in the workplace the therapist evaluated the barriers and challenges for Ms Zelasnik in performing her work, as well as the opportunities for making enhancements. Thus the focus of the evaluation and recommendations was centred in Ms Zelasnik's work place. In this setting, the management was openly supportive of workstation redesign and the need to make improvements in the work environment to accommodate her needs. The employer, her uncle, was in favour of making things easier as he recognised her to be an extremely valuable employee and member of the team.

Analysing work occupations

Ms Zelasnik has primary responsibility for the financial records and for purchasing items in the store. She also takes orders from the business contractors and private individuals who come into the store. Tasks associated with ordering glass include keeping stock up-to-date and tracking the inventory. Ms Zelasnik usually works a 40-hour week. About 20 hours of each week she spends sitting at the front desk with the various tasks of answering the phone, working with customers, using the till and working on the computer, keeping the financial and order records. The other 20 hours she is on her feet, walking through to check orders in the back storage room and making sure that everything is where it needs to be.

On a daily basis, Ms Zelasnik interacts with two other employees who cut some of the custom glass, wrap the glass to be picked up by customers, and do much of the heavy lifting. All three employees, including Ms Zelasnik, take turns working at the front desk to help customers who come into the store or place orders by phone, fax or the internet. Mr Zelasnik, the owner, oversees the work, goes to trade shows to determine if there are new products that he should carry, hires new employees and takes care of managerial issues.

After completing the worksite visit, the therapist described the work environment, characterising the workplace atmosphere as both supportive and pleasant for the employees. While Mr Zelasnik expects high standards of work, he is also flexible about work times and provides time off when needed by his employees. All of the current employees indicated that they enjoyed the work, liked their employer and subsequently have stayed with the company for the past 5 years.

At the end of the chapter, there will be questions related to Ms Zelasnik's occupations. Think about her and her occupational needs as you read about ergonomics and the role of occupational therapy in this area of work.

FUNDAMENTAL CONCEPTS FOR UNDERSTANDING ERGONOMICS

- *ANSI:* This is the American National Standards Institute.
- *Anthropometry:* Anthropometry is the study of the dimensions of people. Anthropometric values may be obtained from populations and applied to the individual or may be acquired directly from the individual.
- *CSA:* The Canadian Standards Association (CSA) determines many different types of standards, including electrical standards and work standards, in Canada.
- *Ergonomics:* Ergonomics is the study of the relationship between the workplace and worker. It is also related to workplace design and equipment adaptations or changes that enhance the work environment with the intention of reducing the incidence and severity of work-related difficulties.
- *Human factors:* Research in the area of human factors is the science of designing the interface between the worker and the environment.[3]
- *ISO:* This is the International Standards Organisation.
- *MSD:* Musculoskeletal disorder. The National Institute for Occupational Safety and Health (NIOSH) replaced the term cumulative trauma disorder with the term musculoskeletal disorder. MSD is an umbrella term that indicates a gradual onset physical disorder related to repetitive activities, to static work in uncomfortable positions, or to a stressful work environment.[4]
- *NIOSH:* This is the National Institute for Occupational Safety and Health in the USA.
- *OSHA:* The Occupational Safety and Health Administration is a regulatory body in the USA.

EVALUATING WORKPLACE DEMANDS

A number of methods are used to evaluate workplace design. The tests can include questionnaires,[5] objective observations,[6] worksite anaylsis,[7–9] simulation,[10,11] videotaping with further analyses,[12] computer training,[13,14] and modelling.[15,16] Most professionals document observations and measurements on a worksite analysis form, commonly referred to as a physical or job demands analysis form.

There is a suggestion that the prevalence rates of risk factors identified through questionnaires are around double those evaluated using a combination of questionnaires and physical examinations. This finding does not mean that questionnaires alone should be used by therapists. It suggests that therapists who want to find out about general problems with a particular work environment need to consider that the prevalence of a particular problem may only be half of what is reported. There is strong support for carrying out a physical examination or evaluating the workplace alongside looking at the results of questionnaires.

Epidemiological studies of injuries and other aspects of the worker and the work environment are important and useful for the therapist to read and understand. They provide guidelines about the possibility of injuries. They do not, however, provide information about how a worker may respond to specific risk factors found in the workplace.[17]

Biomechanical models and studies conducted in laboratories do not replace epidemiological studies, but they provide additional information to help us understand the complex combination of risk factors that may result in injury or disease. Hence, manufacturers are now using ergonomic information in the design and development of products, to create tools or equipment more suited to human capacity. These tools provide a better match for the needs of the user.

Worksite evaluations of risks and hazards using core ergonomic principles are becoming more commonplace. Employers often employ therapists with ergonomic training to assist in workstation redesign and injury prevention in the workplace. Identifying biomechanical and other confounding risk factors in the workplace, through onsite work analysis while workers are performing tasks, leads to a more in-depth understanding of job-specific problems. Understanding the interplay of impairments arising from risk factors of the work itself, or those attributed to the manner in which work is performed, can assist in the early prevention of problems that otherwise may lead to injury and occupational disruption for workers.

DEMANDS OF WORK OCCUPATIONS

Occupations exert both physical and psychological demands on workers. The physical demands were traditionally thought of in terms of hard physical work with lifting. However, there has been an increase in understanding the demands on the less physically active worker. Figure 8.2 shows how two people can easily be involved in accomplishing the same goal in different ways and with different demands. Figure 8.2b shows someone using heavy equipment to dig a trench, while Figure 8.2a shows another person doing the same job by hand. What type of injuries might occur over the long term if these two individuals were to do these tasks daily over many years? Sedentary workers can become injured by repeating the same postures and activities many times. This section will address some of the demands of work occupations.

Physical demands

All work environments entail physical demands. Some of these physical requirements do not cause problems for workers, others may not cause problems to the average worker but may produce difficulties for some workers,[18] while some jobs may actually cause difficulty for most people who attempt to do the work.[19] Pain, as a sequel to injury, is related to

Figure 8.2   Digging a trench.

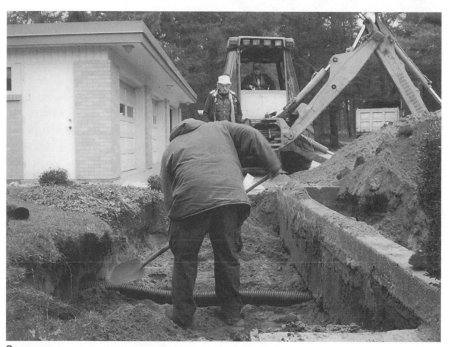

a

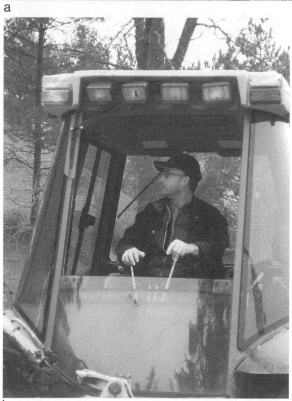

b

reduction of quality of life.[20] Sometimes it is not only the physical demands, but also the cognitive and behavioural demands, along with the complex social interactions with others, that contribute to work discomfort. Demands of work occupations also vary by the nature of the work, for example whether it be heavy or sedentary, across industry sectors.

Heavy industry

The work demands of heavy industry are extensively researched because there are many known risk factors associated with heavy work. These include factors such as carrying heavy loads that may cause injury to the person doing the lifting and standing,[21] working surfaces,[22] and time when tasks are performed in the working day.[23] Current guidelines for acceptable loads that people can lift are available through national safety standards associations such as NIOSH, or through government agencies such as the Ministry of Labour. Methods for lifting using proper body mechanics or mechanical lifting devices that can reduce the chances of back injuries for workers are also available. Mechanical lifting devices are often recommended to reduce the strain on body structures that can lead to injuries. Knowing how to use heavy devices safely in the workplace is equally important (see Fig. 8.3). At Workright Inc. the emphasis is on educating workers on the safe use of equipment and the use of body mechanics when moving heavy loads. Injured workers get an opportunity to put knowledge into practice before returning to work. Consider a shorter

Figure 8.3 Training for lifting: using a mechanical device.

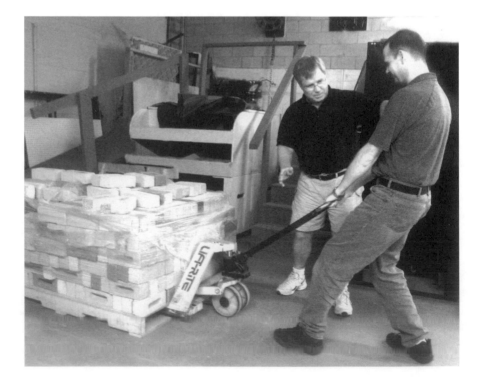

person moving the same skid of bricks (see Fig. 8.3). What, if any, are the important ergonomic considerations to include in the training process? Training packages can be obtained through workplace health and safety training agencies.

Sedentary work

In the current century, many people have sedentary occupations, many of which involve working at a computer or video display terminal (VDT).[24] Some full-time VDT users complain of many physical upper extremity problems.[25] For example, Hsu & Wang[26] found that the prevalence of upper extremity complaints was 42% for full-time VDT users. The authors did suggest, however, that scheduling of working hours and breaks is important in designing VDT jobs. Other researchers have also evaluated the relationship between breaks and work during VDT use and found that well-designed breaks may be useful.[27] Researchers provide ergonomic recommendations for children who use computers at school,[28–31] and others[32–34] evaluate methods of teaching office ergonomics.

It appears that finger forces used during keyboarding work are higher than actually required to push down the keys. Arm supports can alleviate strain[35] and reduce muscle activity in some of the back muscles. Also, the actual muscle activity as measured by electromyography may be low, but this does not imply that there may not be upper extremity problems.

Computer use often requires the individual to use peripheral devices, such as a computer mouse. A variety of these peripheral devices are available to computer users, with some of the devices being advertised as 'ergonomically designed'. The therapist can be in a quandary when asked to recommend a mouse or a specific keyboard design. One researcher[36] did a kinematic study of hand and upper extremity movements with two different pointing devices. The findings of the study determined that with two very different pointing devices, there was a similarity in performance. Individuals had minimal movements with either device. This finding suggests that individuals who use a computer pointing device for much of their computer use could be prone to having difficulties as a result of prolonged static hand and upper extremity positions.[37] Another study recommends the use of a case study based on a CD-ROM to help students learn about the ergonomic issues found in work stations.[38]

Computer work spaces

The computer era has led to the rapid evolution of a new area of ergonomics over the past few years. New problems have arisen from using computers and working in sedentary activities, which were not apparent in the age of heavy work environments. Such problems include seating postures that, if uncorrected, can lead to back and neck related problems. Many people multitask while using a computer, for example using a head set to answer the phone, searching for information on the computer, or recording information by hand. Together, these tasks add to the types of strains, such as eyestrain and headaches, that individuals can experience through prolonged exposure. There are also potential problems associated with using a keyboard for great lengths of time without a break. One common problem is carpal tunnel syndrome. Many occupational therapists who work in the area of hand therapy or ergonomics find their clients have had carpal tunnel releases. These individuals not only need post-surgery therapy, but may also need environmental changes to reduce the possibility of other work-related injuries occurring.

Evaluating and redesigning workstations to promote function and reduce risks is a collaborative process. Figure 8.4 shows an ergonomic specialist and an injured person working together to explore adjustments for improving productivity and managing risks associated with computer workstations. Note the elevation of the monitor to align vision and promote functional neck postures while performing computer tasks. Here, the worker is trialling a natural keyboard intended to reduce wrist deviation while typing. In addition, a forearm support is used to reduce arm and shoulder strain while working at a workstation for long periods of time. What other tasks and equipment are used in conducting work on a computer? What types of adjustments could you recommend to improve functioning and comfort for persons who use a computer for more than 4 hours a day?

Cognitive and behavioural demands

There is a growing interest in examining and evaluating the cognitive and behavioural demands of work occupations,[39] such as decision-making, degree of supervision, or social interactions with others required to manage

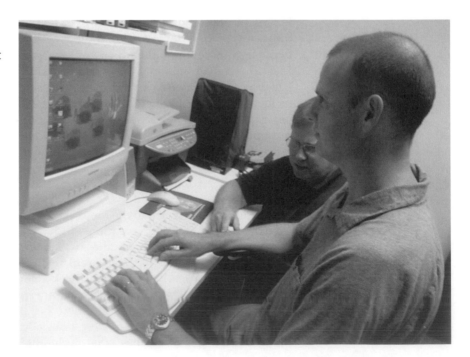

Figure 8.4 Working together to reduce risks at the workstation at Workright Inc., London, Ontario.

conflicts of customers or co-workers. Expanding job analysis beyond the physical demands is necessary due to the interplay of the effects of stressors in heightening the tension in muscles required to perform manual tasks. If left unaddressed, the influence of potentially stressful work demands that require intensive concentration, multitasking or decision-making under pressure, can also lead to lost productivity for workers due to headaches, ulcers and mental health concerns. In addition, people's perceptions of the meaning and relevance[40] of their work may add to productivity problems and discomfort experienced. A thorough discussion of the psychosocial factors associated with work is beyond the scope of this text, but it is very important. Studies are finding that the psychosocial aspects of work can be related to the physical difficulties that may be experienced at work.[27]

Demands of the work environment

Most worksite evaluations take into account environmental considerations that may add to the risk to people in performing their work. These considerations include the effect of repetitive lifting in cold areas or of working in noisy workplaces where hearing protection may be mandated. Beyond these physical aspects of the work environment, there are numerous other areas that need to be part of the process of evaluating risks. Work performance is affected by many factors, including the impact of rotation, team processes, collective agreements and shift work, in addition to work procedures and rules put in place for the benefit of workers and employers, to meet safety requirements. These aspects of the work environment need to be taken into account when identifying barriers and challenges to making changes. Healthy employment relationships and social support from co-workers and employers can also lead to a positive workplace atmosphere, where workers feel not only a sense of connectedness, but also have greater freedom to suggest and implement improvements to work processes. On the other hand, workplace atmospheres that are not viewed as supportive can pose challenges for therapists and workers in their attempts to make ergonomic improvements. More research is needed to assist therapists in understanding how to address system or cultural barriers in the workplace.

ERGONOMIC PRINCIPLES IN (RE)DESIGNING WORK OCCUPATIONS OR THE ENVIRONMENT

When designing a work environment many aspects of the environment must be considered, including lighting, temperature, ventilation, work heights, tool design, reach area of the workers,[41] and many other factors. Often ergonomists, who may have training in kinesiology and/or engineering, are involved in such designs. Their level of training suggests that they would be the appropriate experts for this type of work. However, when a person with a pre-existing injury or disability is planning to enter or re-enter the workforce, an occupational therapist is a valuable person to have on the team. Occupational therapists' understanding of physical problems, the recovery process, and workplace adaptations, as well as their focus on meeting the individualised needs of specific clients, can offer insights into the occupational and environmental strategies needed for effective work re-entry programmes.

One of the purposes of designing the work environment is eliminating predisposing factors to injury. For example, researchers have found an increase in hand lacerations if individuals are asked to rotate between jobs where concentration and precision work with sharp instruments is required.[42] On the other hand, rotation of job tasks can reduce boredom and length of exposure to more physically demanding tasks, such as are found in assembly lines in automotive plants. In addition, the expense must be considered when adapting environments. It is often less expensive to change the environment before an injury occurs, than to wait until compensation and rehabilitation of workers is necessary, and subsequently incur additional expenses associated with workstation redesign. Some researchers suggest that there is a cost benefit to ergonomic work.[43] Involving the worker in the work place evaluation can also be effective in identification of problems.[44–46]

Anthropometric considerations

Anthropometry, specifically data that determine the average physical characteristics of a worker, has been used in the design of equipment for specific occupations. The problem with depending solely on average anthropometric information is that most people are not 'average', so tools, workstations or heavy equipment designed this way will not necessarily fit everyone, and may in fact be detrimental to some individuals. The problem with using anthropometric data is compounded when we consider the people whom occupational therapists help. Not only do these people frequently not meet anthropometric averages, they usually also have special needs in relation to the work environments and occupations they perform.

Force considerations

Forces in the environment can cause problems for workers. These forces include, but are not limited to, shear, compression and tension. If any of these forces are too high, beyond the maximal capacity of a person, injury can occur. For example, if a person who uses a wheelchair for mobility needs to do a sliding transfer to a chair that has a rough surface in order to work, he could end up with skin breakdown due to the shear force between his skin and the rough surface.

Lifting very heavy loads repeatedly can cause compression of discs between the vertebrae. Excessive or repeated loadings can also cause injury to joint structures such as articular cartilage. Osteoarthritis can be a long-term consequence of cartilaginous deterioration.[4] Tension can also cause damage, for example to a person with compromised tendons who tries to slow down a moving object by pulling on it.

Strength considerations

Manual strength is important when considering the use of tools in the workplace. Differences are noted in maximum obtainable hand-grip force, depending on different upper limb positions. Grip strength is an index of hand power and the maximum obtainable hand-grip is thought to help predict hand function. Maximum force in grip strength can be affected not only by different upper arm positions, but also by the person's occupation, standing or sitting posture, the diameter of the grip, the type of measuring tool[47] or dynamometer that is used, nationality, lifestyle, body mass and age. Some work has been conducted to evaluate hand-tools and determine a method to design the tools ergonomically, so that they fit the task.[48]

Dexterity and gripping

Pinching and grasping can be done in a variety of postures and some of these postures may predispose individuals for upper extremity problems. For instance, positioning is important. The load on the muscles is lowered when the fingers can wrap around an object using a power grip. On the other hand, muscle loading can easily be tripled during trigger forces if a bent wrist is used as opposed to a straight wrist.[49]

Vibration and friction in tool design

Equipment vibration that is not damped or attenuated causes stress on joints, muscles and tendons. In addition, exposure over the long term to low-frequency vibration of tools can injure arteries or constrict blood flow.[3] Tools should be adapted to keep the vibration to a minimum. This vibration absorption can be accomplished by adding padding to the equipment or providing the worker with gloves that offer some damping of the vibration and protection from over exposure.

There are other mechanical principles that should be considered when looking at human functioning and optimal use of equipment. A high coefficient of friction between a piece of equipment and a person's hand or glove will decrease the chances of slipping. For example, if a person were using a pair of pliers to do electrical work, it would be important for the person to have a grip that would not slip. A tool should weigh as little as possible within safety standards so that stress or fatigue is not precipitated by the tool use. Often therapists or kinesiologists can offer workers and employers insights into the purchase of tools and equipment that support comfort and reduce potential for injury.

Participatory ergonomics

The implementation and application of ergonomic principles in the workplace must involve employers providing the resources necessary for making physical changes in the work environment. Its success is also reliant upon worker involvement. Worker involvement is crucial in putting into practice key principles of safe lifting, and disseminating knowledge to minimise personal exposure to unnecessary risks. Participatory ergonomics includes workers in the process of implementing ergonomic knowledge and encourages management support for workers to make adjustments or changes to reduce physical risks.[50] Research has demonstrated that participatory ergonomics involving workers, unions and employers is effective in early return to work for workers with low back pain arising from manual work tasks.[51] Thus, optimal success in either injury reduction or safe and timely return to work can be achieved through increasing worker involvement in and knowledge of ergonomics. Therapists and kinesiologists need to share information about their individual expertise in ergonomics and to encourage collaboration. They also need to encourage application of principles by all work place parties.

DEMANDS AND ERGONOMIC CONSIDERATIONS OF INDIVIDUALS PERFORMING WORK: FACTORS RELATED TO THE INDIVIDUAL

There are many factors relating to the individual concerned that need to be considered when making recommendations for design or redesign of workstations or work processes. Personal risk factors for overuse disorders are thought to include age, female gender, previous trauma, diabetes, rheumatoid arthritis, wrist size or shape, and hormonal factors. Common work activities, such as gripping and pinching, may produce significant tension in the finger flexor tendons. For instance, assembly plants that hire predominantly female workers need to consider purchase of hand tools that offer workers a variety of smaller grip sizes to optimise performance and reduce exposure to risks associated with gripping. Occupational factors that may put a person at risk include jobs that involve repeated or sustained exertions,[52] forceful exertions, awkward postures, contact stresses, dynamic effects of hand motions, and the work organisation. It is important for the therapist to be aware of the interplay of personal and occupational risk factors in making recommendations for workplace change and in the design of return-to-work programmes for persons recovering from musculoskeletal disorders.

Older workers

A current trend in many workplaces is the hiring and retention of older workers. This poses a new concern for professionals and employers, i.e. dealing with the physical and cognitive changes of workers who are aging. Present demographic trends mean that there are and will continue to be more older workers. One of the growing concerns about older workers who remain in the workforce longer, is the potential for more work-related injuries, or other problems associated with aging that may predispose them to being injured in the workplace. A review of the literature on aging suggests that the physical decline associated with a decreased reaction or response time is the biggest concern for accommodating the older worker.[53] Another issue that could present a problem for older workers is the rapidly changing workplaces of today. This adds a level of uncertainty for the worker. Although dealing with uncertainty is not a problem solely for the older worker, change could be an issue for these individuals. A better understanding of the important applications of biomechanical principles in relationship to older workers is needed.

People returning to work after a work-related or non-work-related physical problem

People returning to work following an injury or disabling incident have many issues with which to contend.[54] They may not be able to return to their previous position or may have to adapt their occupations or environments so that they can return to work. Furthermore, persons experiencing an occupational disruption from work due to physical injury are often anxious about their abilities and the potential for re-injury upon resumption of pre-injury job tasks.

The occupational therapist and/or the kinesiologist should be involved in this transition from an injury or a rehabilitation programme to a return to work programme. Occupational therapists and kinesiologists can work in collaboration with clients and employers to suggest changes to the work environment or tools that make it easier for a person to perform work tasks.

A key part of the training of occupational therapists, however, is in identifying accommodations and opportunities. Therapists involve individuals in managing their own impairments. They also determine what is needed to facilitate recovery and confidence in work functioning for persons with permanent and progressive disabilities. Research indicates that programmes of rehabilitation are found to have increased effectiveness if motivation is enhanced during the rehabilitation.[55] Hence, involving the worker in informed decision-making on recovery strategies, and in taking on an active role in using ergonomic principles in performing work as part of the rehabilitation process, may lead to a more timely and safe return to work.[56]

People entering the workforce who have a physical disability

Individuals who have chronic illnesses[57] or physical disabilities often want to enter the workforce[58-60] or return to work. Occupational therapists help people with physical problems to overcome barriers to entering the workforce.[61] Initially, the therapist helps to determine the type of work a person can perform. The therapist may also go into a workplace to help adapt the environment. These adaptations, if needed, are functionally designed, so that a person with a disability will successfully conduct job tasks. Assistance and professional support can be helpful to someone who has a disability.[60,62] For instance, Barrett[63] suggests that for some people with severe impairments, personal assistants are needed to enable them to conduct work that is meaningful. In other cases, job coaches or co-worker mentors can be valuable in helping a person with a disability, who requires a longer period of adjustment, make the transition into work.[64]

SUMMARY

The nature of work is changing rapidly. The physical characteristics and needs of the worker should be considered and taken into account in these changes. Therapists who have a working understanding of the ergonomic concepts discussed in this chapter will be able to help people adapt to work situations and engage in meaningful work activities.

QUESTIONS BASED ON THE CASE

1. What is the primary issue Ms Zelasnik wants the occupational therapist to help her to solve?
2. What are some of the environmental characteristics that are important for Ms Zelasnik? What assessment would you use, if you were the occupational therapist, to determine the environmental characteristics and whether or not they fit her requirements? What do you think will be some of the environmental characteristics that you can change, but still make the workspace useable by others?
3. What aspects of Ms Zelasnik's physical abilities seem to be causing her problems? Are there others that you might want to ask her about or to assess in your consideration of possible changes?
4. It appears that Ms Zelasnik's occupations are difficult for her. How would you assess some of these occupations and what suggestions might you make? You can make assumptions about her occupations, in order to consider changes.
5. The accommodations you would recommend must not interfere with other people's ability to work in the environment. How would you accomplish this part of the therapist's role?
6. What ergonomic principles might be useful in evaluating the occupations and the work environment? How would these principles be used by the therapist in recommending changes to the workplace? How could these principles be used by Ms Zelasnik to promote optimal work performance on a daily basis?
7. There are a number of internet websites related to work issues. If you have access to the internet, try to find these websites. Are some of them better than others? Be very careful in evaluating the sites you choose to use for assessment and treatment information.

Laboratory Exercise: Examples of Ergonomics

The purposes of this exercise are:
1. To evaluate your own work environment. You will determine if there are factors in your environment that may be enhancements to your work. You will also try to determine any characteristics of your work that could be altered using ergonomic principles.
2. To take the information about your working environment and see if it would be manageable by a person who is using a wheelchair. You will determine what, if any, adaptations you would make to the environment that would make it easier for a wheelchair user to find the environment effective.

To begin the exercise, you should collect some anthropometric data about yourself. Measure and record the following parameters, or have another person measure them for you: your arm length, leg length, total body height, length of body from seat to the top of your head when you are sitting down.

Now you should go through your average work day. You will want to document some of the activities mentioned below as you go through the day. These are only some of the occupations that you may be engaged in. If there are other important occupations, be sure to document them as well. You might also want to consider videotaping some of your movements if you think that they might be important, but they are difficult to describe.

Some of the occupations to document:
1. Method of travel to your work setting. For example, if you walk to work, how long does it take? What type of surface do you walk on, pavement or gravel? What are the usual weather conditions? Do the weather conditions change during the year and if so, how does that affect your ability to get to work? Do you carry anything with you? If so, how do you carry it and how much does it weigh?
2. Once you are in your work setting, evaluate your environment. Do you have to go up stairs? What is the lighting like? What is your workspace like? Remember to consider issues such as desk height, table height and any other measurements of the environment that affect how you conduct your work.
3. Document each of the occupations that you do during your day. How long do you do them? Are there any heavy work activities that you do? Do you sit and make notes? How long do you sit, without a break? What is your workplace layout, seated workstation height and what are some of the pieces of equipment that you routinely use?
4. What other activities are you engaged in during your workday? Document any activities that you do during the day related to your occupation.

Once you have documented your work occupations and environments, consider carefully if there are aspects of them that might be changed to help prevent potential work-related problems or fatigue.

Occupational therapists who work with individuals with acquired or congenital physical problems can be in the position of helping someone adapt or accommodate their occupations and/or environments. To have an opportunity to practise thinking about some possible adaptations, consider the implications of participating in your daily work occupations while using a wheelchair for mobility. How would using a wheelchair affect your daily activities? What aspects of your occupations would you have to adapt? Are there any occupations that you would have to abandon completely? Is the environment functional for someone who uses a wheelchair? How will using a wheelchair affect the speed at which someone can move around the environment? Will the wheelchair dimensions affect the ability of the person to work? Will there be a change in the person's envelope of reach?

Try to find and examine a current assessment form, from your learning environment, clinical community, national occupational therapy association or a website, that is designed to consider issues related to wheelchair users and work, and that can give you some ideas about how to adapt the environment and one's occupations for the person in a wheelchair.

As you do this laboratory exercise, consider any other physical difficulties that might interfere with someone's work.

USEFUL WEBSITES

http://stats.bls.gov
http://www.cdc.gov/niosh/homepage/html

REFERENCES

1. Wilson JR. Fundamentals of ergonomics in theory and practice. Appl Ergon 2000; 31(6):557–567.
2. Shaw L, Polatakjo H. An application of the occupation competence model to organizing factors associated with return to work. Can J Occup Ther 2002; 69(3):158–167.
3. Warren N, Sanders M. Biomechanical risk factors. In: Sanders M, ed. Ergonomics and the management of musculoskeletal disorders. 2nd edn. St Louis: Butterworth Heinemann, 2004:191–229.
4. Dillon C. Joint injury and arthritis in the spectrum of workplace MSDs. In: Sanders M, ed. Ergonomics and the management of musculoskeletal disorders. 2nd edn. St Louis: Butterworth Heinemann, 2004:132–148.
5. Redfern MS, Chaffin DB. Influence of flooring on standing fatigue. Hum Factors 1995; 37(3):570–581.
6. Clasby RG, Derro DJ, Snelling L, Donaldson S. The use of surface electromyographic techniques in assessing musculoskeletal disorders in production operations. Appl Psychophysiol Biofeedback 2003; 28(2):161–165.
7. Hanson CS, Shechtman O, Gardner-Smith P. Ergonomics in a hospital and a university setting: the effect of worksite analysis on upper extremity work-related musculoskeletal disorders. Work 2001; 16(3):185–200.
8. Peper E, Wilson VS, Gibney KH, et al. The integration of electromyography (SEMG) at the workstation: assessment, treatment, and prevention of repetitive strain injury (RSI). Appl Psychophysiol Biofeedback 2003; 28(2):167–182.
9. Schulze LJ, Delclos GL, Pinglay N. Integrated job analysis: a technique to document job activities and to identify occupational risk factors and modes of remediation and accommodation. Int J Occup Environ Health 2001; 7(3):222–229.
10. Nussbaum MA, Chaffin DB. Effects of pacing when using material handling manipulators. Hum Factors 1999; 41(2):214–225.
11. Nussbaum MA, Chaffin DB, Stump BS, et al. Motion times, hand forces, and trunk kinematics when using material handling manipulators in short-distance transfers of moderate mass objects. Appl Ergon 2000; 31(3):227–237.
12. Hanse JJ, Forsman M. Identification and analysis of unsatisfactory psychosocial work situations: a participatory approach employing video–computer interaction. Appl Ergon 2001; 32(1):23–29.
13. Feyen R, Liu Y, Chaffin D, et al. Computer-aided ergonomics: a case study of incorporating ergonomics analyses into workplace design. Appl Ergon 2000; 31(3): 291–300.
14. Robertson MM, Amick BC III, Hupert N, et al. Effects of a participatory ergonomics intervention computer workshop for university students: a pilot intervention to prevent disability in tomorrow's workers. Work 2002; 18(3):305–314.

15. Mallis MM, Mejdal S, Nguyen TT, Dinges DF. Summary of features of seven biomathematical models of human fatigue and performance. Aviat Space Environ Medicine 2004; 75(3):A4–A14.
16. Rosen J, Arcan M. Modeling the human body/seat system in a vibration environment. J Biomech Eng 2003; 125(2):223–231.
17. Dekker SW. Accidents are normal and human error does not exist: a new look at the creation of occupational safety. Int J Occup Saf Ergon 2003; 9(2):211–218.
18. Dempsey PG, McGorry RW, O'Brien NV. The effects of work height, workpiece orientation, gender, and screwdriver type on productivity and wrist deviation. Int J Ind Ergon 2004; 33(4):339–346.
19. Craig BN, Congleton JJ, Kerk CJ, et al. A prospective field study of the relationship of potential occupational risk factors with occupational injury/illness. AIHA J: a Journal for the Science of Occupational & Environmental Health & Safety 2003; 64(3):376–387.
20. Andersen JH, Kaergaard A, Frost P, et al. Physical, psychosocial, and individual risk factors for neck/shoulder pain with pressure tenderness in the muscles among workers performing monotonous, repetitive work. (Including commentary by Riihimaki H.) Spine 2002; 27(6):660–667.
21. Konz SA, Rys MJ. An ergonomics approach to standing aids. Occup Ergon 2002; 3(3):165–172.
22. Simeonov PI, Hsiao H, Dotson BW, Ammons DE. Control and perception of balance at elevated and sloped surfaces. Hum Factors 2003; 45(1):136–147.
23. Lombardi DA, Sorock GS, Hauser R, et al. Temporal factors and the prevalence of transient exposures at the time of an occupational traumatic hand injury. J Occup Envir Med 2003; 45(8):832–840.
24. Smith MJ, Bayehi AD. Do ergonomics improvements increase computer workers' productivity? An intervention study in a call centre. Ergonomics 2003; 46(1–3):3–18.
25. Korhonen T, Ketola R, Toivonen R, et al. Work related and individual predictors for incident neck pain among office employees working with video display units. Occup Environ Med 2003; 60(7):475–482.
26. Hsu W, Wang M. Physical discomfort among visual display terminal users in a semiconductor manufacturing company: a study of prevalence and relation to psychosocial and physical/ergonomic factors. AIHA J: a Journal for the Science of Occupational & Environmental Health & Safety 2003; 64(2):276–282.
27. Baker NA, Jacobs K, Tickle-Degnen L. The association between the meaning of working and musculoskeletal discomfort. Int J Ind Ergon 2003; 31(4):235–247.
28. Bennett CL. Computers in the elementary school classroom. Work 2002; 18(3):281–285.
29. Rowe G, Jacobs K. Efficacy of body mechanics education on posture while computing in middle school children. Work 2002; 18(3):295–303.
30. Shinn J, Romaine K, Casimano T, Jacobs K. The effectiveness of ergonomic intervention in the classroom. Work 2002; 18(1):67–73.
31. Williams CD, Jacobs K. The effectiveness of a home-based ergonomics intervention on the proper use of computers by middle school children. Work 2002; 18(3):261–268.
32. Bohr PC. Office ergonomics education: a comparison of traditional and participatory methods. Work 2002; 19(2):185–191.
33. Leonard-Dolack DM. The effectiveness of intervention strategies used to educate clients about prevention of upper extremity cumulative trauma disorders. Work 2000; 14(2):151–157.
34. Richardson D. Ergonomics and retention. Caring 2002; 21(9):6–9.
35. Lintula M, Nevala-Puranen N, Louhevaara V. Effects of Ergorest arm supports on muscle strain and wrist positions during the use of the mouse and keyboard in work with visual display units: a work site intervention. Int J Occup Saf Ergon 2001; 7(1): 103–116.
36. Merla JL. An electromyographic and kinematic comparison of two computer pointing devices. MSc Thesis. The University of Western Ontario, London, Canada: 1998.
37. Putz-Anderson V. Cumulative trauma disorders: a manual for musculoskeletal diseases of the upper limbs. Philadelphia: Taylor and Francis; 1988.
38. August-Dalfen S, Snider L. A multimedia case based approach to the study of office ergonomics. Work 2003; 20(1):3–11.

39. Raybould K, McIlwain L, Hardy C, Byers J. Improving the effectiveness of the job demands analysis tool. Toronto: Occupational Health and Safety and Workers' Compensation Board; 1999.

40. Shaw L, Segal R, Harburn K, Polatakjo H. Understanding return to work behaviours: promoting the importance of individual perceptions in the study of return to work. Disabil Rehabil 2002; 24(4):185–195.

41. Kozey JW, Das B. Determination of the normal and maximum reach measures of adult wheelchair users. Int J Ind Ergon 2004; 33(3):205–213.

42. Bell JL, MacDonald LA. Hand lacerations and job design characteristics in line-paced assembly. J Occup Envir Med 2003; 45(8):848–856.

43. Beevis D. Ergonomics – costs and benefits revisited. Appl Ergon 2003; 34(5):491–496.

44. Motamedzade M, Shahnavaz H, Kazemnejad A, et al. The impact of participatory ergonomics on working conditions, quality and productivity. Int J Occup Saf Ergon 2003; 9(2):135–147.

45. Rosecrance JC, Cook TM. The use of participatory action research and ergonomics in the prevention of work-related musculoskeletal disorders in the newspaper industry. Appl Occup Environ Hyg 2000; 15(3):255–262.

46. Westgaard RH. Work-related musculoskeletal complaints: some ergonomics challenges upon the start of a new century. Appl Ergon 2000; 31(6):569–580.

47. McGorry RW. A system for the measurement of grip forces and applied moments during hand tool use. Appl Ergon 2001; 32(3):271–279.

48. Aptel M, Claudon L, Marsot J. Integration of ergonomics into hand tool design: principle and presentation of an example. Int J Occup Saf Ergon 2002; 8(1):107–115.

49. Moore A, Wells R, Ranney D. Quantifying exposure in occupational manual tasks with cumulative trauma disorder potential. Ergonomics 1999; 34(12):1433–1453.

50. Nagamachi M. Requisites and practices of participatory ergonomics. Int J Individ Ergon 1995; 15:371–377.

51. Loisel P, Gosselin L, Durand P, et al. Implementation of a participatory ergonomics program in the rehabilitation of workers suffering from subacute back pain. Appl Ergon 2001; 32:53–60.

52. Nahit ES, Taylor S, Hunt IM, et al. Predicting the onset of forearm pain: a prospective study across 12 occupational groups. Arthritis Care Res 2003; 49(4):519–525.

53. Gillin EK, Salmoni A, Orange JB, et al. When is a worker too old to work? [Unpublished manuscript. 2004.]

54. Taimela S, Diederich C, Hubsch M, Heinricy M. The role of physical exercise and inactivity in pain recurrence and absenteeism from work after active outpatient rehabilitation for recurrent or chronic low back pain: a follow-up study. Spine 2000; 25(14):1809–1816.

55. Gardt G, Larsson A. Focus on motivation in the work rehabilitation planning process: a qualitative study from the employer's perspective. J Occup Rehabil 2003; 13(3):159–167.

56. Strong S, Shaw L. Client-centred ergonomics. In: Jacobs K, ed. Client-centred ergonomics. Boston: Butterworth Press.

57. Martin DJ, Brooks RA, Ortiz DJ, Veniegas RC. Perceived employment barriers and their relation to workforce-entry intent among people with HIV/AIDS. J Occup Health Psychol 2003; 8(3):181–194.

58. Riches VC, Green VA. Social integration in the workplace for people with disabilities: an Australian perspective. J Vocation Rehab 2003; 19(3):127–142.

59. Sokka T. Work disability in early rheumatoid arthritis. Clin Exp Rheumatol 2003; 21 (5 Suppl 31):571–574.

60. Turner E. Using a personal assistant in the workplace. J Vocation Rehab 2003; 18(2):81–85.

61. Gilworth G, Chamberlain MA, Harvey A, et al. Development of a work instability scale for rheumatoid arthritis. Arthritis Care Res 2003; 49(3):349–354.

62. Strobel W, McDonough JT. Workplace personal assistance service and assistive technology. J Vocation Rehab 2003, 18(2):107–112.

63. Barrett JC. Being an effective workplace personal assistant. J Vocation Rehab 2003; 18(2):93–99.

64. Pentland W, Drummond H. Coaching: what does it offer you and your clients? Occup Ther Now 2004; 610–612.

Chapter 9

Leisure for people with disabilities

Leisure is important for everyone. There are times when we need to re-energise, relax, enjoy ourselves, or spend time with others in a non-work environment. Leisure is as important for people who have physical difficulties as it is for anyone else. Some of us do not focus much on leisure during our training to become therapists. Sometimes we do not give it the credit it is due nor do we always address it during therapy once we are working. We may not include it in our work with people because time is taken by seemingly more pressing matters, such as the person returning home or going back to work. There does not seem to be much emphasis on evaluation of leisure activities, working with people to make their leisure time more meaningful for them, or helping people to choose activities they want to do.

Leisure time can encompass participating in sports and other physical activities, reading, spending time with friends, or participating in any number of different activities. Some people like to be involved in activities directly related to their cultural backgrounds. Figure 9.1 shows a man participating in Highland Games, which originated in Scotland. Think about any specific activities that are culturally relevant for you, and consider if they could be adapted so that people with physical disabilities could participate. Recreational activity does not always require highly technical equipment. The boy in Figure 9.2 is enjoying rolling a tyre in the schoolyard.

Figure 9.1 Highland Games.

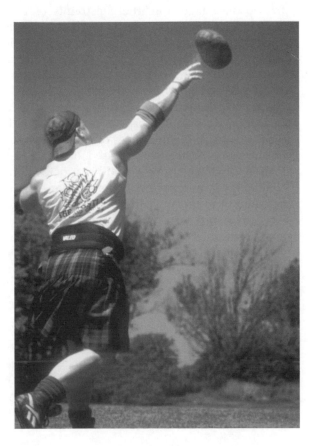

Figure 9.2 Having fun with a tyre.

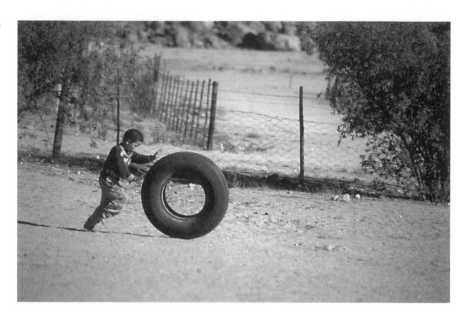

He is balancing both the tyre and himself, so he is getting good physical exercise while having fun. The individuals with whom we work should be free to disengage from the constraints of real life and enjoy leisure as everyone else does. Schleien[1] notes the importance of having choices and being free from responsibilities for people with disabilities. It has been suggested by a number of authors that individuals with disabilities who do not participate in leisure activities will spend a great deal of time unoccupied during their lifetime.[2]

This chapter will encourage the reader to consider some of the issues related to leisure in respect to people with physical problems and disabilities. The biomechanics of sports in relation to people with physical disabilities will not be discussed directly, as this is addressed in other texts.[1,3–6] Following a case study of a person with physical disabilities, the chapter gives an overview of the components of various physical activities. In addition to physical difficulties, other difficulties, such as hearing and intellectual problems will be mentioned, as these can be barriers to the enjoyment of leisure that need to be overcome. Training and participation, and issues of accessibility, are also discussed.

Before reading the rest of the chapter, please read the following case thoroughly. Then, after reading on, think about how some of the information in the chapter may be used to help Melanie Matthews.

CASE STUDY: MELANIE MATTHEWS

Melanie is a 12-year-old girl who is in her first year of junior high school. She has spina bifida and uses either a wheelchair or a walker to get around. She prefers to use a wheelchair when she is in a hurry, but likes to use the walker for exercise. She wants to participate more fully in her regular class's physical education programme than she has in past years. The class has a well qualified physical education instructor, Ms Carruthers, who is eager to work with Melanie.

The setting

The setting is the junior high school. The building is wheelchair accessible, as are both the gym and the outdoor playing fields. The school has a number of students who have physical problems.

The occupational therapist

The occupational therapist, Mr Joseph Barts, has been working as a school-based occupational therapist for about 5 years. He is interested in helping pre-teens and teenagers become involved in activities. He has worked in camps for children with multiple disabilities, has actively coached many teams, and is a qualified swimming instructor. He has been working with Melanie since she was 7 years old.

The individual

Melanie lives with her parents and two older brothers in an apartment. Both of her parents work and her two brothers go to the same high school that she started at this year. The family enjoys sports and have included Melanie in their activities. They swim at a local pool. They also like horseriding and though it is expensive for them, they manage to get out on a few weekends every year to a place not far from the city where the children take lessons and do trail riding. Melanie has been involved in a riding programme for children with disabilities and really enjoys it.

She has had spina bifida since birth. She is lacking neural input to her legs, but she has very strong arms. She does not have the cognitive problems that sometimes accompany spina bifida. She does, however, have some difficulty concentrating for long periods of time. Though her concentration span is less than that of her peers, she tries to compensate by working hard at school.

Physical abilities

Melanie's arms are very strong and her hands have normal dexterity. She uses a wheelchair for mobility, although she can get in and out of it herself and crawl for short distances. She also uses a walker to go short distances. Her problem is that she has very little function in her legs.

She uses a catheter for urination, which she manages on her own during the day at school. She is on a bowel programme which does not interfere with her school activities.

Emotional and intellectual status

Melanie is a kind, outgoing girl, who makes friends easily. She is at a cognitive level equal to her peers. She is used to having spina bifida, but does not like the fact that her friends can go faster than she can. She is also starting to be self-conscious at high school because she uses a wheelchair and a walker. It is typical for girls to feel unsure of themselves at her age, but she is finding it more difficult than most students usually do.

Exploring issues with Melanie

When helping Melanie set goals for her school year, the occupational therapist found that Melanie's hope is that for physical education she will be able to move from the class designed for children with special needs to the group which her classroom friends attend. Like most girls her age, she wants to fit in with friends.

Melanie feels like she is starting to fall behind her brothers in sports. This probably would have happened whether or not she had spina bifida, because they are both older than she is. It is just difficult for her and she would really like to be able to do more on her own, without the family.

Leisure activities for Melanie

Melanie, the occupational therapist, and the physical education instructor have decided to meet during the year to assess Melanie's skills and help determine activities in which she can participate. The occupational therapist will help Melanie develop some physical skills and work with her concentration. Both skills and concentration are required to be involved in the sports she wants to join.

The first issue is to determine the sports that are suitable for Melanie to join. She can consider wheelchair sports as well as ones that are with her other school friends.

Fitness

Involvement in physical activities promotes fitness. Individuals who have physical difficulties may be more at risk of being unfit than people who do not have these problems. This is one reason why individuals with such problems should be encouraged by their therapists to consider physical activities as part of their leisure programme. Research has suggested that young people with cerebral palsy, muscular dystrophy, or visual impairments lead comparatively sedentary lifestyles relative to youths with other types of impairments, including physical, chronic medical or hearing problems.[7] Researchers have found that African-American women with severe disabilities have very low levels of physical activity, and that this exposes them to risk of secondary health conditions.[8] Individuals with Parkinson's disease appear to benefit both physically and psychologically from exercise training.[9]

Graham and Reid[10] have carried out research on the physical fitness of adults with intellectual disabilities. They found that over time adults with intellectual disabilities are more at risk than the general population for declining health in relation to low physical fitness and aging. Improved physical performance among a population of individuals with intellectual disabilities demonstrated that these people were able to successfully participate in and benefit from physical activity and performance.[10] These authors provide information about very diverse groups of people with specific difficulties, both physical and intellectual. Their research findings serve to remind us of the importance of considering leisure and fitness with the people with whom we work.

Attitudes

When discussing participation in leisure activities, it is important to consider the attitudes of both the individuals wanting to participate, and their peers. Positive attitudes towards involvement can help to ensure that the leisure activity is enjoyable for individuals. Research has been conducted into the behaviours of individuals involved in leisure activities. Fenning et al[11] found that sportsmanship behaviours of a basketball clinic's participants did not differ between participants with and those without a disability. There appeared to be an increase in the understanding of individual differences and sportsmanship on the part of the adolescents involved.

Research[12] has shown that women with disabilities manage their disabilities in different ways and may have different attitudes towards physical activities such as sport and exercise. They may see themselves as either able or unable to engage in such activities, and some may minimise the significance of the body, so that it is not particularly important to them. Therapists should take into account how the women they work with see themselves, and may have the opportunity to challenge a woman's perception of her abilities. Other authors found that participating in wheelchair basketball leads to improved physical abilities and physiological function for female athletes who have experienced spinal cord injuries.[13]

Therapists should consider suggesting activities that promote physical fitness as leisure pursuits when appropriate. They should think about how the people they work with could be introduced to such activities. They also need to discuss the possible attitudes of others and how negative attitudes might be handled, if they are voiced.

Assessments

Biomechanists analyse activities either qualitatively or with extensive use of equipment. Biomechanical assessments of movements can be useful when considering any leisure activities that include physical components. Biomechanical analyses of gait or posture can provide information about the basic movements a person can carry out. Other assessments can also be used to provide information to the therapist who is helping someone to decide on and learn new physical skills.

Analysing a task encompasses identifying all the component skills and sequences, and considering appropriate interactions with the activity and with other players.[1,14] This analysis, properly done, will help in creating successful leisure experiences for the individuals concerned. Schleien[1] describes a task analysis form that can be used to determine the components and requirements of a leisure activity. It has a format recommended for use with students with complex disabilities. Any assessment the therapist chooses and any recommendations the therapist makes to encourage sports and leisure participation should include all of the following:

- cover multiple measures of function
- observe activities within the context in which the child or adult will be involved
- be accompanied by programming ideas
- focus on the skills needed for the child to become an independent adult
- focus on function rather than form.

It has also been suggested that a clear link between assessment and intervention goals should be established.[15]

A number of motor fitness tests are available. The tests have been designed for professionals who work with individuals with motor difficulties. Some of these tests are listed in Box 9.1, and the reader should consider which of them will be useful for helping Melanie.

Unfortunately, low fitness scores tend to occur for some individuals with intellectual disabilities, when these tests are administered. These low scores may not simply reflect the person's disability, they may be an indication of lack of quality of instruction, lack of opportunity to practise, as well as the physical characteristics or the medical complications of the individual.[16]

Cratty[17] suggests that assessments should contain evaluation of the objectives for the programme as well as its components. Lack of agreement between the stated objectives, the evaluation and the programming could lead to disappointment or frustration for the people involved. It has been suggested by Schleien et al[18] that evaluating data may be a waste of time if the results are not shared with the individuals involved in the programme. The authors suggest that unless the consumers of the services, their family, and agency management receive the information from evaluations, results may not be useful.

Box 9.1   Some motor fitness tests

1. The Project Transition Assessment Test. Obtained from Dr Paul Jansma, The Ohio State University Department of Physical Education, 343 Larkin Hall, Columbus, Ohio, 43210.
2. Kansas Adapted/Special Physical Education Test Manual. Obtained from Janet Wilson, Specialist in Physical Education, Kansas State Department of Education, 120 E 10th Street, Topeka, Kansas, 66612.
3. Bruininks–Oseretsky Test of Motor Proficiency. Obtained from the Amercian Guidance Service, Circle Pine, Minnesota, 55014.
4. Data-Based Gymnasium. Obtained from PRO-ED Publishers, 5341 Industrial Oaks Boulevard, Austin, Texas, 78735.
5. Special Olympics Inc. Sports Skill Instruction Program Manual. Obtained from Suite 500, 1550 NY Avenue, NW, Washington DC 20005

TRAINING AND PARTICIPATION

Training and participation are both essential to any therapy plan and implementation. People who are trained well can enjoy an activity with more self-confidence than those who have had no training. The training itself can be done in groups, allowing interaction with other people. Training programmes that are used for everyone diagnosed with a particular disability, regardless of individual differences, may be ineffective. People with disabilities should have individually tailored programmes that are age suitable and based on personal interest. For example, Melanie should be helped by the therapist to find an age-specific programme for a sport she enjoys, as she is keen to be involved with people her own age. Her participation in such training will probably help her to feel better about performing her chosen sport or activity.

Principles of motor control and learning can be applied when working with people who have physical disabilities. Therapists can become trainers or instructors in a particular activity or sport if they have current knowledge of the skills involved in that activity.

Once information about a person's interests and abilities has been obtained, intervention can be evaluated for its effectiveness. A multidisciplinary approach to working with an athlete with physical disabilities may be appropriate, because each profession involved will have a unique contribution to make.[19] Once information about a person's interests and abilities has been obtained, participation options can be discussed. The goal would be to find activities that fit with the individual's enjoyment and fitness interests. A multidisciplinary approach may be appropriate. For example, kinesiologists, coaches familiar with particular sports and therapists might all be involved in a fitness programme. The kinesiologists and coaches or instructors might provide the background and expertise in instruction for specific activities. Therapists might aid the success of the programme by providing information about issues related to the person's physical problems. In some situations, instructors may have special training to work with people with disabilities, and the only role of the therapist might be to help an individual find such an instructor.

Specific sports programmes have been examined to determine their effectiveness for people with disabilities. Traditional learn-to-swim progressions may not be appropriate for most children with physical disabilities.[20] This would suggest that programmes designed specifically for these children may be more effective in helping them learn to swim. The therapist should consider the availability of such programmes and trained instructors when discussing involvement in sports programmes.

People who have learning disabilities may have specific needs that present challenges. Cognitive difficulties may occur with or without physical problems. These intellectual challenges must be met if an individual is to become successfully involved in a leisure programme. For example, emotionally disturbed children may exhibit behaviours that make it difficult for them to learn. It is important to help these individuals manage their behaviours.[14] The behaviours may spill over into the area of leisure and should be addressed there, too. A child who is displaying inappropriate behaviours will have difficulty fitting in with any activity group, so it would be appropriate for a therapist to help with addressing such behaviours before a programme of activity begins.

Individuals with orthopaedic difficulties present a challenge to physical educators and occupational therapists. Orthopaedic difficulties can occur at any time. A problem may be present at birth, or happen later in life. The therapist needs to take the orthopaedic difficulties into account and may be involved in explaining any adaptations or precautions that must be taken for an individual. Therapists must also consider any medical restrictions that might apply to people with orthopaedic problems. Occupational therapists may help the physical educator to adapt either the activities or the environment, or both, to deal with orthopaedic restrictions.[14]

Effective communication is essential during training, regardless of the abilities of the learner. The requirements of communication may need to be adapted by teachers of individuals who have hearing difficulties. The instructor should concentrate on all of the following:

- the position of the learner with respect to the teacher
- the intensity of commands
- any hearing aids used by the learner
- the environment in which learning is occurring.[14]

Visual impairment and loss of vision have implications for motor, intellectual, social and psychological development. The purpose of physical activity for individuals with visual difficulties is for enjoyment, as it is with other people. Physical activity will improve both motor and social skills for people with visual limitations. It is considered appropriate to create environments with support systems and people who can facilitate participation.[14] Although designing environments is not always possible, it may be important to facilitate participation by individuals in other ways.

An occupational therapist who is familiar with working with people with difficulties and who is aware of environmental design issues, may be involved in designing the environment or making recommendations for adapted sports facilities. The therapist who is involved in environmental adaptations should think about some of the issues about the environment raised in this chapter, and should, if possible, incorporate universal design. In designing accessible environments, helping individuals to choose activities, and ensuring that there is a good fit between the leisure skills and the person, the occupational therapist will have an important contribution to make in promoting fitness and encouraging leisure activities.

INJURIES

Occupational therapists may work with athletes who have disabilities and subsequent sports related injuries. When dealing with any type of injury the therapist must consider the person who has been injured, the occupation that was performed, and the environment in which it was performed. The therapist may be able to intervene in these areas and, using understanding of movement and the mechanical principles behind the movement, change the conditions so the person may return to the activity.

Although sports injuries are well researched, injury trends in people who have disabilities are not well documented. Research needs to be carried out in this area so that programmes for injury prevention can be established.

A number of injuries have been determined as needing to be addressed by an occupational therapist. For example, shoulder and upper extremity pain in women wheelchair basketball players is extremely common and should be addressed by healthcare providers, coaches, and players.[21] Wheelchair use can result in shoulder pain. In one study, 72% of subjects reported shoulder pain since beginning wheelchair use and 52% reported current shoulder pain. The results of this study suggest the importance of individuals and their coaches and healthcare professionals addressing the prevention of pain and chronic disability in individuals who use wheelchairs.[21]

PARTICIPANT INVOLVEMENT

Often, individuals with disabilities spend a great deal of time not engaged in activities.[1,6] They may not have the skills to be involved in play or leisure activities, nor be in contact with people with whom they can participate.[1] They often need lifelong assistance.[6] The occupational therapist should consider this when recommending leisure activities. It would be ideal, for example, to find activities that Melanie can learn now, that she will also be able to do when she is older. Swimming, an activity she already does, is a good sport for her to carry on through her life. There may be other sports or activities that work in this way for her, but this will not always be the case and is not absolutely necessary, because many people do change the sports and activities in which they participate throughout their lives.

FAMILY INVOLVEMENT

Families are often the first recreation delivery system. We do not always think of a family in that way, but if the family members are active, it is usually the first place a child who has physical challenges learns his or her skills. Then it is important to move beyond the family situation to consider separately both the needs of the individual with disabilities and the needs of other members of the family.[18] This is the situation for Melanie, who wants to continue being involved in family activities, but also wants to do more with friends her own age. The therapist working with her, then, is working in more than one environment. The therapist must consider the environments of the home, the school and the larger community. The recreational and social needs of the entire family must be considered when involving participants in a programme.

PROFESSIONAL INVOLVEMENT

Traditionally, motor, communication and social skills were taught separately, whereas now they may be taught in conjunction with one another and with other skills, and their teaching is often embedded within ordinary curricular activities, including sports.[15] They may also be taught in sports facilities. However, we also need to remember that many children participate in sports without adults teaching them, and with an emphasis on fun, not just skill development.

The transdisciplinary approach seems to be the most effective method of training.[14] There are three major steps the therapist and special educator may require to take to implement this approach:

- First, the therapist should understand the special educator's job or role.
- Second, the therapist should have knowledge of the roles of other specialists who may work in schools.
- Third, the special educator should have a variety of strategies to work most effectively with other specialists to meet student needs.[22]

Integrating students with special needs is important, so they can feel part of their peer group. It appears that using a special physical educator to help integrate a child with cerebral palsy into a kindergarten physical education class is very effective. A case study suggested the child in this situation was accepted socially and was successful in motor participation.[23] People with special needs may even be able to participate in some extreme sports; for example people who are unable to use their lower extremities may still be able to participate in sports requiring upper extremity strength, such as whitewater kayaking. Figure 9.3 shows people doing an Eskimo roll to right themselves after being submerged in the water. Are there any reasons why people with physical problems should or should not be involved in extreme sports?

Figure 9.3   Whitewater kayaking.

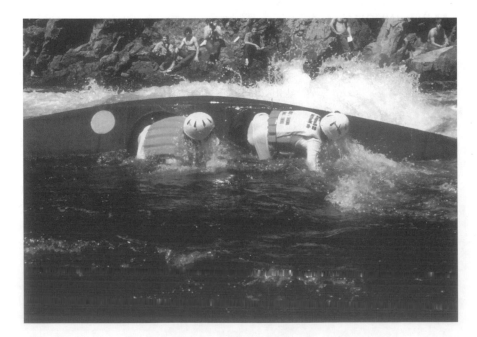

It is possible for an occupational therapist to discover the motivations that might lead to an individual participating in a particular leisure pursuit. The therapist can also help people find new activities to replace those activities they can no longer participate in.[24] A commitment to making choices and enjoying leisure activities can have lifelong implications, and this should be considered carefully during the planning of leisure activities.[18]

Therapists may provide both direct and indirect therapy. This means that they may either work directly with the individual who wants to participate in an activity, or they may help other members of the team, including physical educators, to design programmes for individuals. For example, they may teach the teacher or other members of the team to integrate particular strategies and methods into a child's preschool activities to help ensure success.[15]

Occupational therapists may also offer the traditional services of assessment and treatment for individuals with serious disabilities. Their areas of concern will include fine motor functioning skills and perceptual motor programmes, activities of independent living, and monitoring uses of adaptive devices which have been designed to enhance independence.[25] Therapists will be aware that the participation in activities of the people they work with may be modified through adaptation of rules, materials or task sequences.[1] The occupational therapy programme will be designed to assist individuals to obtain maximum independence by minimising the impact of their disabilities.[16]

ATHLETIC TRAINING

People with physical difficulties participate and compete in sports at all levels. Those who are involved in elite athletics need to train using many of the same methods that are used by anyone who needs to prepare for competition. Top-class athletes with disabilities need a wide variation in training programmes. Harlick and McKenzie[26] suggest, following an extensive review of the literature of sports psychology, that the mental skills training programmes typically used by developing athletes should be available to athletes with disabilities. The unique needs of athletes with disabilities should be considered. Improvements in coaching and training for many of these elite-level athletes are essential, so they can compete to the best of their abilities just like any other elite athlete.[27]

TRAINING FOR PEOPLE WITH LEARNING DIFFICULTIES

This text is designed for the therapist working with people who have physical difficulties. Sometimes physical difficulties, depending on the diagnosis and also on the individual, can be accompanied by other difficulties such as learning or concentration problems. These problems should not stop most people from being involved in leisure activities. Many people who have learning difficulties do extremely well when they are physically active. Occupational therapists should not dismiss sport and leisure pursuits as possible activities for individuals who have such difficulties.

There are issues the therapist should consider when working to help someone with a learning difficulty participate. Individuals with learning difficulties cannot always spontaneously adopt effective strategies during motor tasks.[28] It appears, however, that providing precise visual information for some people with learning difficulties will increase their skills in some areas, for example their throwing accuracy.

Balance is one area that can be usefully addressed for some individuals with learning difficulties. Woolacott and Shumway-Cook[29] suggest that individuals with Down syndrome cannot rely, during posture, on a feedforward control process as used by typically developing children. They tend to rely more upon a feedback strategy for controlling the interaction between voluntary systems and posture. Successful training for these individuals can be accomplished by:

- increasing the complexity of the environment
- progressing from reducing redundancy of sensory inputs to increasing sensory complexity.

This increase in the complexity of the environment may result in functional improvement in balance for these children.

Reaction times of individuals who have mild intellectual disabilities appear to be slower than those of people with average intellectual skills. This reduced response time may indicate that information processing mechanisms are somewhat different from those in individuals who do not have intellectual difficulties.[30] This slowing appears in simple motor tasks. It may result from the process of response initiation at the beginning of a motor act.[31] Some suggestions for cognitive skill training include:

- knowing your domain
- knowing your learner
- training in multiple contexts
- giving directed feedback
- instructing in generalised action
- providing instruction in self-management
- training in the environment in which the activity takes place.[32]

One success story is that of the Special Olympics, which have grown from a very small start to being the largest and most visible organisation for sports that are specifically for individuals with learning disabilities.[16]

CLASSIFICATION OF ATHLETES

A classification system has been designed for athletes, so that an individual will compete with people who have similar abilities. Occupational therapists who are trained in assessing the level of ability in individuals can become involved in helping people determine which is the appropriate classification for their participation in sports competitions. Fairness in grouping individuals for sports participation is an issue[33] that is addressed by trying to ensure people will compete with other people who are at a similar level of function.

Athletes with disabilities are classified according to their physical, intellectual and emotional abilities, and they compete against other people who have similar abilities. In this way, the training and skill level of the individual becomes the most important factor in the competition.

Classification can be medically, functionally, or performance-related. Because classification may be based on three different sets of criteria, an individual athlete with a serious disability may be put into a level of competition to which they may be unable to respond, physically or psychologically.[6]

ACCESSIBILITY ISSUES

Occupational therapists who have an understanding of biomechanics are in a position to alleviate problems of accessibility for individuals. Therapists will make it easier for participation to occur if they help individuals by eliminating the barriers to participation.

Barriers to participation

Individuals with disabilities experience environmental barriers to participation in and access to sports competitions.[6] Other external barriers to participation may include financial constraints, lack of accessible facilities, poor communication, ineffective service systems, negative attitudes and lack of qualified staff.[18] An occupational therapist with an understanding of leisure pursuits and some knowledge of mechanics will be able to have an impact on reducing environmental barriers.

Another barrier to participation is found in individuals themselves. For example, some individuals who have learning difficulties may have movement difficulties or cardiovascular endurance problems. This lack of endurance impacts on movements skills and may preclude these individuals from participating in many physical activities.[16] Other individual barriers are skill limitations, health, lack of knowledge of activities, and dependence on others.[18]

Physical accessibility

Architectural barriers limit the ability of people to participate. Some of the features which may make it difficult to participate include:

- inaccessible travel routes to activities
- ground surface characteristics within a facility
- bathroom facilities that may be inadequately adapted
- showers that are inaccessible
- lack of detectable warning and alarm systems.[18]

Venues for activities

Leisure activities can take place in a variety of places, from an adapted playground to international sports venues. Athletes can participate in sports at many levels, from the recreational to the highly competitive and elite.

Integration

'Least restrictive environments' describes non-institutional service approaches to activities for people with physical difficulties. Using a least restrictive environment approach suggests that people involved with leisure instruction want this leisure to occur in typical community environments.[18] A number of intervention strategies to encourage inclusive recreation have been described by Schleien et al.[18] Some of the strategies include:

- structuring the environment to encourage cooperation and peer-to-peer interaction
- preparing peers who are not disabled to be cooperative companions and tutors to individuals who are
- creating a team
- adapting tasks to promote access while implementing skill training for individuals with disabilities.

There is an attempt to encourage people with disabilities to use community resources, rather than having them participate in segregated environments.[18,34] Individuals with moderate or severe learning disabilities have traditionally been excluded from community recreation programmes and have been involved, whenever involvement occurred, in segregated programmes.[35] Jansma et al[6] suggest that, using a functional skills curriculum, the key is to conduct an inventory of alternatives for skills which the individual needs. The authors suggest that individuals may need the skills to function in their current and projected environments, specifically a community centre.

Integration must become a reality. Inclusion of young people with disabilities in leisure activities appears to be enhanced if young people with and without disabilities are in contact on a regular basis. This inclusion is most likely to occur if accommodations are minimal and occur naturally, and if equal status and relationships occur.[36]

There are a number of benefits noted for people with disabilities integrating into the community setting. Children without disabilities may serve as role models during activities for individuals who have problems. The opposite may also occur, with the children with disabilities becoming the role models. An added benefit is that by playing in a community setting, children are actually involved in the settings in which the activities most appropriately occur. Integrating students into mainstream education may affect group dynamics, relationships, teachers and instructors.

If individuals have leisure interests that correspond with their skills, these abilities may allow them to participate in community settings.[1] A playground which is well-designed enhances the natural environment and offers opportunities for play for individuals with different abilities in mobility.[37] Generally, there are very few, if any, reasons to exclude people with physical and intellectual problems from the community.

Legislation

Legislation can facilitate the inclusion in the community of people with physical problems. Occupational therapists do not need to know biomechanical principles to promote inclusion; however, if the inclusion is based on constructing environments and determining the needs of people with physical disabilities, the occupational therapist needs an understanding of movement to promote useful legislation. An example of including individuals with disabilities in leisure activities is provided in the USA, where it is mandatory for parks and recreation services to be accessible, though other limitations, including inaccessible facilities and lack of staff training, may make it difficult for individuals to participate.[38] Consider your own country. Is there legislation in place that promotes the inclusion of individuals with physical problems in leisure and sports activities where you live? Where you live, how can you make your knowledge of a person's movement abilities and of the environment impact on positive legislation for people with physical problems?

SUMMARY

People often have leisure time: time to participate in activities they enjoy. Participation for people who have difficulties can require some adaptations of the environment and extra training on the part of the staff who are working in the area of leisure. The importance of leisure activities is underscored by the number of assessments available and the legislation, in different jurisdictions, to encourage participation. Occupational therapists interested in helping someone to be involved in leisure activities have many resources available to them, so they can encourage individuals in making leisure skills an integral aspect of their lives.

QUESTIONS BASED ON THE CASE

1. What activities might be appropriate for Melanie to try? What adaptations would need to be made for the activities that you are considering? Also consider activities for Melanie that may need no adaptations.
2. What precautions should Melanie take to reduce the chance of injuring herself?
3. What role does the occupational therapist have in helping Melanie meet her goals?
4. If Melanie is unsuccessful with a sports activity at school, what should be done? If that happens, who should be involved in future decisions about Melanie's involvement in the athletic curriculum at the school?

continued overpage

5. Should Melanie's classmates be informed about Melanie's involvement and what should they be told?
6. Are there any assessments that the occupational therapist should carry out with Melanie before she becomes involved in physical activity classes?
7. Who are the other members of the transdisciplinary team who would be involved in helping Melanie participate in leisure activities?

Laboratory Exercises

1. Consider your family environment when you were 12 years old. If you were a child who used a wheelchair for mobility, but had no other difficulties, what sort of leisure activities would you have tried? What might have been some of the barriers for you? Where would you have liked to participate in these activities: your home, school, or community?
2. Find a community facility, such as the Young Men's Christian Association (YMCA), in the town in which you live. Is it accessible for someone who uses a wheelchair? If not, what would make it accessible? Are there any special programmes that are designed specifically for individuals who are unable to participate in regular programmes? Are there programmes that could be adapted for people with intellectual disabilities? Are there programmes that individuals with physical disabilities could join, without any adaptations being made to the programmes?
3. Consider that you are being required, as an occupational therapist, to help a recreation therapist design a leisure programme for older individuals who all have a visual difficulty called macular degeneration. This is a vision problem in which the central field of vision does not function well. The person can see movement, but usually cannot see colours and cannot read. What leisure activities might be appropriate for this person? How would you determine which activities you and the recreation therapist might try with the person?
4. Choose assessments and a training programme for a 10-year-old child who has Down syndrome, assuming that the child has 6 months to prepare for participation in a track and field programme that is designed for children with learning difficulties.
5. Identify 10 activities that would be age-appropriate for people with spasticity and minimal function of the lower extremities. Think of activities for people who are: 5, 15, 25, 35, 45 and 60 years of age. Assume that each person uses a walker for ambulation, has good use of the upper extremities, and has no intellectual or emotional difficulties.
6. Evaluate the requirements for a leisure programme that lends itself to life-long participation.
7. Formulate a plan to determine the physical barriers of a major amateur or professional sports venue that is in your home town, or near it.
8. Find out what your legal legislation is for involving people with physical problems in activities.

REFERENCES

1. Schleien SJ. Lifelong leisure skills and lifestyles for persons with developmental disabilities. Baltimore: PH Brookes; 1995.
2. Jansma P. Psychomotor domain training and serious disabilities. 5th edn. Lanham: University Press of America; 1999.
3. Lieberman LJ, Cowart JF. Games for people with sensory impairments: strategies for including individuals of all ages. Champaign: Human Kinetics; 1996.
4. Steadward RD, Wheeler GD, Watkinson EJ. Adapted physical activity. Edmonton: University of Alberta Press; 2003.
5. Davis RW. Inclusion through sports. Champaign: Human Kinetics; 2002.
6. Jansma P, Wallstrom T, Walsh M. Psychomotor domain training and serious disabilites. In: Jansma P, ed. Psychomotor domain training and serious disabilities. 5th edn. Lanham: University Press of America; 1999:101–130.
7. Longmuir PE, Bar-Or O. Factors influencing the physical activity levels of youths with physical and sensory disabilities. Adapted Physical Activity Quarterly 2000; 17(1):40–53.
8. Rimmer JH, Rubin SS, Braddock D, Hedman G. Physical activity patterns of African-American women with physical disabilities. Med Sci Sports Exerc 1999; 31(4): 613–618.
9. Reuter I, Engelhardt M, Stecker K, Baas H. Therapeutic value of exercise training in Parkinson's disease. Med Sci Sports Exerc 1999; 31(11):1544–1549.
10. Graham A, Reid G. Physical fitness of adults with an intellectual disability: a 13-year follow-up study. Res Q Exerc Sport 2000; 71(2):152–161.
11. Fenning P, Parraga M, Bhojwani V, et al. Evaluation of an integrated disability basketball event for adolescents: sportsmanship and learning. Adapted Physical Activity Quarterly 2000; 17(2): 237–252.
12. Guthrie SR. Managing imperfection in a perfectionistic culture. Quest 1999; 51(4):369–381.
13. Schmid A, Huonker M, Stober P, et al. Physical performance and cardiovascular and metabolic adaptation of elite female wheelchair basketball players in wheelchair ergometry and in competition. Am J Phys Med Rehabil 1998; 77(6):527–533.
14. Auxter D, Pyfer J, Huettig C. Principles and methods of adapted physical education and recreation. 9th edn. Blacklick: McGraw-Hill; 2001.
15. Gallivan-Fenlon A. Integrated transdisciplinary teams. In: Jansma P, ed. Psychomotor domain training and serious disabilities. 5th edn. Lanham: University Press of America; 1999:29–36.
16. Eichstaedt CB, Lavay BW. Physical activity for individuals with mental retardation. Infancy through adulthood. 5th edn. Champaign: Human Kinetics Books; 1992.
17. Cratty BJ. Adapted physical education in the mainstream. 2nd edn. Denver, CO: Love; 1989.
18. Schleien SJ, Ray MT, Green FP. Community recreation and people with disabilities: strategies for inclusion. Baltimore: PH Brookes; 1997.
19. Lai AM, Stanish WD, Stanish HI. The young athlete with physical challenges. Clin Sports Med 2000; 19(4):793–819.
20. Gelinas JE, Reid G. The developmental validity of traditional learn-to-swim progressions. Adapted Physical Activity Quarterly 2000; 17(3):269–285.
21. Curtis KA, Black K. Shoulder pain in female wheelchair basketball players. J Orthop Sports Phys Ther 1999; 29(4):225–231.
22. Lavay B, French R. The special physical educator: meeting educational goals through a transdisciplinary approach. In: Jansma P, ed. Psychomotor domain training and serious disabilities. 5th edn. Lanham: University Press of America; 1999:19–28.
23. Vogler EW, Koranda P, Romance T. Including a child with severe cerebral palsy in physical education: a case. Adapted Physical Activity Quarterly 2000; 17(2):161–175.
24. Bonder RR, Wagner MB. Functional performance in older adults. Philadelphia: FA Davis; 2001.
25. Kimble K, Ball B, Jansma P. Role of the physical therapist and occupational therapist: addressing serious disabilities. In: Jansma P, ed. Psychomotor domain training and serious disabilites. 5th edn. Lanham: University Press of America; 1999:67–74.

26. Harlick M, McKenzie A. Psychological skills training for athletes with disabilities: a review. New Zealand Journal of Sports Medicine 2000; 28(3):64–66.

27. Liow DK, Hopkins WG. Training practices of athletes with disabilities. Adapted Physical Activity Quarterly 1996:372–381.

28. Davis WE. Precise visual information and throwing accuracy of mentally handicapped subjects. In: Wade MG, ed. Motor skill acquisition of the mentally handicapped. Amsterdam: Elsevier Science; 1986:25–44.

29. Woollacott MH, Shumway-Cook A. The development of the postural and voluntary motor control systems in Down's syndrome children. In: Wade MG, ed. Motor skill acquisition of the mentally handicapped. Amsterdam: North-Holland; 1986:45–72.

30. Zelasnik HN, Aufderheide SK. Attentional and reaction time analysis of performance: implications for research with mentally handicapped individuals. In: Wade MG, ed. Motor skill acquisition of the mentally handicapped. Amsterdam: Elsevier Science; 1986:45–72.

31. Karrer R. Input, central and motor segments of response time in mentally retarded and normal children. In: Wade MG, ed. Motor skill acquisition of the mentally handicapped. Amsterdam: Elsevier Science; 1986:167–187.

32. Brown AL, Campione JC. Training for transfer: guidelines for promoting flexible use of trained skills. In: Wade MG, ed. Motor skill acquisition of the mentally handicapped. Amsterdam: Elsevier Science; 1986:257–272.

33. Daly DJ, Vanlandewijck Y. Some criteria for evaluating the 'fairness' of swimming classification. Adapted Physical Activity Quarterly 1999; 16(3):271–289.

34. Kozub FM, Zelms L. Community-based high school physical education model. In: Jansma P, ed. Psychomotor domain training and serious disabilities. 5th edn. Lanham: University Press of America; 1999:181–194.

35. Pollinque H, Cobb H. Leisure education: a model facilitating community integration for moderately/severely mentally retarded adults. In: Jansma P, ed. Psychomotor domain training and serious disabilities. 5th edn. Lanham: University Press of America; 1999:242–252.

36. Wilhite B, Devine MA, Goldenberg L. Perceptions of youth with and without disabilities. Ther Recreation J 1999; 33(1):15–28.

37. Raschke C, Dedrick C, Hanus K. Adaptive playgrounds for all children. In: Jansma P, ed. Psychomotor domain training and serious disabilities. 5th edn. Lanham: University Press of America; 1999:483–494.

38. Devine MA, Kotowski L. Inclusive leisure services: results of a national survey of park and recreation. Journal of Park and Recreation Administration 1999; 17(4):56–72.

Index

Page references to non-textual material such as Boxes, Figures or Tables are in *italic* print